SEX ED IN THE DIGITAL AGE

DIGITAL AGE

Volume 2

By

Carolyn Cooperman, MA, MSW

Edited by

Susan Milstein, PhD, MCHES, CSE

Copyright © 2014 by
The Center for Sex Education
196 Speedwell Avenue, Morristown, NJ 07960
(973) 387-5161
www.SexEdCenter.org

ISBN: 978-1-941843-01-7

*This manual was produced with generous support from contributors to
The Center for Sex Education, the national education division of
Planned Parenthood of Central and Greater Northern New Jersey, Inc.*

ABOUT THE AUTHOR

CAROLYN COOPERMAN, MA, MSW has worked to promote sexual health as both an educator and therapist. For Planned Parenthood affiliates, she provided teacher training, parent education and curriculum assistance to multiple school districts throughout northern New Jersey. She co-authored the original versions of *New Methods for Puberty Education* with Chuck Rhoades, MA, PhD, and *Positive Images: A New Approach to Contraceptive Education* with Peggy Brick, MEd. While working with Planned Parenthood, Carolyn organized a sexual abuse clearinghouse for information, referral and prevention education. Her experience as an educator also includes teaching introductory human sexuality courses at Nassau Community College, and both undergraduate- and graduate-level teacher training courses at Fairleigh Dickinson University, Florham/Madison Campus. Carolyn was a senior staff member at a community-based agency servicing individuals and families. She provided educational workshops for parents who were in the process of adapting to blended families. Her areas of specialization in clinical practice include treatment for the effects of infertility, sexual abuse, marital problems, chronic illness and women's issues.

ABOUT THE EDITOR

SUSAN MILSTEIN, PhD, MCHES, CSE is a professor in the Department of Health Enhancement at Montgomery College in Maryland. She has taught there for fourteen years, and is the resident "sexpert" for the "Ask the Sexpert" seminar for students. She is also part-time faculty at George Washington University. Susan also provides sexuality education for people of all ages through Milstein Health Consulting (www.milsteinhc.com). In addition to her media appearances and national and international presentations, she has worked on many teaching manuals including the award-winning *Teaching Safer Sex, 3rd Ed.; Positive Images: Teaching about Contraception and Sexual Health* and *Changes, Changes, Changes: Great Lessons for Puberty Education.* Susan is the director of education and outreach for the Woodhull Sexual Freedom Alliance.

CONTRIBUTING AUTHORS

Meghan Benson

Kirsten deFur

Margo DeNuccio

Catherine Dukes

Shanna M. Dusablon Drone

Ashley Gaunt

Josefina Gil-Leyva

Christine L. Hackman

Lee Heerten

Corbin Knight-Dixon

Susan Milstein

Holly Moyseenko

Hannah M. Priest

Karen Rayne

Rebecca Roberts

Sarah E. Rush

Timaree Schmit

Jessica Shields

Jessica Silk

Bill Taverner

ACKNOWLEDGMENTS

We would like to take this opportunity to thank the following people who contributed to the development and publication of *Sex Ed in the Digital Age*:

The Planned Parenthood of Greater Northern and Central New Jersey (PPCGNNJ) Board of Directors, whose support of sexual health education has allowed the production of many excellent teaching resources.

Nora Wong, who recognized the importance of this manual from the outset. Nora and her husband Raymond provided substantial funding to see this manual published.

Major supporters of The Center for Sex Education (CSE), including **Barbara E. Bunting, Alexandra and Eric J. Schoenberg, Pat Stover, Naida S. Wharton** and **Raymond and Nora Wong,** who for so many years have given generously in support of sexuality education.

Triste Brooks, president and CEO of Planned Parenthood of Central and Greater Northern New Jersey (PPCGNNJ). Few CEOs are as committed to honest, accurate and positively framed sexuality education as Triste.

All of the talented **educators and authors** who developed the creative lessons and resources in these two volumes. See their names on the "Contributing Authors" page.

Mary Lyn Koval, copyeditor, who carefully reviewed the massive manuscript. How fortunate we are to have a friend and colleague who is also an expert copyeditor and passionate supporter of our work!

Kerry E. Mack, who designed the great covers of these manuals.

Jeffrey Anthony, who coordinated the printing, and **Zoe Roselli,** who reviewed the manuscript layout.

Nancy Jenner, Cheryl Wenzinger, and our friends at **McNaughton-Gunn,** who did the print job.

All the experts who critically reviewed the manuscript and/or gave endorsements, including **Megara Bell, Heather Corinna, Brian Flaherty, Osmo Kontula, Elizabeth Mooney, Jack Myers, Cory Neering, Trina Scott, Amy Settele** and **Katherine Suellentrop.**

Melissa Keyes DiGioia, for sharing her knowledge and experience, and providing encouragement.

Joel Cooperman, for his insights and unconditional support during every phase of this project.

Diane Wolfe, who brought her talent as an educator to the review of this manual, and provided invaluable research assistance.

Chuck Rhoades, who generously reviewed lessons and conducted preliminary field testing.

Bill Taverner, for believing in the importance of this project from the outset and securing the necessary funding that allowed it to move forward; showing encouragement and respect in his interactions with the project's many contributors, sometimes putting into words that which was difficult to express; bringing enthusiasm, levity and new direction when needed; and for having the vision to see the tremendous potential in sex education in a rapidly changing world.

And finally, to **sex educators who work directly with teenagers,** we say *thank you* for creating opportunities that allow young people to think critically about the impact of technology on sexuality and relationships.

INTRODUCTION
Teenagers, Technology and Sex

By Carolyn Cooperman, MA, MSW

Sex Ed in the Digital Age was two years in the making. The initial impetus for this project began with an observation that will not come as a surprise to those of us who work in the field of sex education — **teenagers are as interested in technology as they are in sex.** By linking the two, it then becomes possible to tap into an integral part of the adolescent experience. The opportunity to work with young people and explore subject matter that reaches into the core of their development is an exciting prospect for educators.

Today's adolescents have unprecedented access to sexual information. This is a profound change for this generation of teenagers. On their own, without having to wait for parents to purchase books or schools to offer programs, they are bringing their sex-related questions, concerns and interests, and hormone-driven needs, into the technological arena. Modern technology has undone centuries of secrecy surrounding sex. Now it is up to the parents and educators who care about fostering healthy sexual development to bring clarity and purpose to the technological advancements.

These volumes include structured lessons designed to equip educators and parents with skills that are necessary for meeting the challenges of the digital age. The principle objectives of the lessons are to help teens apply discriminating judgment about electronic use; to know how to locate accurate information; and to better understand the impact that electronic communications have on oneself and others.

We are most grateful to sex educators from around the country who wrote lessons for these volumes. Working in middle schools, high schools, colleges and community-based programs, they have a handle on what teenagers are learning about sex from the countless hours that teens spend texting and browsing. Our common goal has been to help adolescents evaluate the appropriateness of their own electronic use.

Bill Taverner, MA, CSE, Executive Director of The Center for Sex Education, played a crucial role in bringing these volumes to fruition. He believed in this project from the outset, contributed original lessons, and set the administrative wheels in motion to make it happen. The editor, Susan Milstein, PhD, MCHES, CSE, significantly enhanced the substance and form of this work. Her attention to detail, background in sex education, and experience in the classroom is truly valued.

PRINCIPLES FOR SEX EDUCATION

Sex Ed in the Digital Age remains faithful to The Center for Sex Education's long-held principles for sex education. It is important for teachers using this edition to recognize these principles and act upon them, since they illustrate basic philosophical and pedagogical approaches to comprehensive sex education. Educators who are mindful of these principles and examples will likely find additional ways to implement them as they teach the lessons.

1 **ALL PARTICIPANTS NEED AND DESERVE RESPECT.** This respect includes an appreciation for the difficulty and confusion of addressing sexual issues and a recognition of the constellation of factors that contribute to those issues. It means treating all persons, both young people and adults, as intelligent individuals who are capable of making decisions in their lives.

2 **PARTICIPANTS NEED TO BE ACCEPTED WHERE THEY ARE.** This means listening and hearing what people have to say, though we as educators might sometimes disagree. In general, we are much better off helping individuals explore the possible pitfalls of their attitudes rather than telling them what they ought to believe.

3 **PARTICIPANTS LEARN AS MUCH OR MORE FROM EACH OTHER AS FROM THE EDUCATOR.** Often, if we let people talk, allow them to respond to each other's questions and comments, and ask for others' advice, they feel empowered and take responsibility for their own learning. It is much more powerful for a participant to challenge a peer's belief or attitude than for the educator to do so.

4 **HONEST, ACCURATE INFORMATION AND COMMUNICATION ABOUT SEX IS ESSENTIAL.** For most of their lives participants may have received messages suggesting that sex is hidden, mysterious and something not to be talked about in a serious and honest way. Limiting what individuals can talk about and using vague terminology perpetuates the unhealthy "secrecy" of sex. Sexual information needs to be presented in an honest, accurate way.

5 **A POSITIVE APPROACH TO SEX EDUCATION IS THE BEST APPROACH.** This means moving beyond talking about the dangers of sex and acknowledging in a balanced way the pleasures of sex. It means associating things open, playful and humorous with sexuality, not just things that are grave and serious. It means offering a model of what it is to be sexually healthy rather than focusing on what is sexually unhealthy.

6 PEOPLE HAVE A FUNDAMENTAL RIGHT TO SEX EDUCATION. They have a right to know about their own bodies and how they function. They have a right to know about any sexual changes that are occurring now and any others that may occur during their lifetimes. They have the right to have their many questions answered. People who have explored their own values and attitudes and have accurate information are in the best position to make healthy decisions about their sexual lives.

7 GENDER EQUALITY AND GREATER FLEXIBILITY IN SEX-ROLE BEHAVIOR HELP ALL PEOPLE REACH THEIR FULL POTENTIAL. These two volumes strongly advocate the right of all people — regardless of their gender — to achieve their full human potential. Strict adherence to traditional gender-role behavior limits people's choices and restricts their potential.

8 ALL SEXUAL ORIENTATIONS AND GENDER IDENTITIES MUST BE ACKNOWLEDGED. The inclusive nature of these lessons recognizes that there are diverse sexual orientations and gender identities, and some participants may identify as lesbian, gay, bisexual, transgender, intersex or questioning. It is important to create an environment that recognizes the needs of these often isolated and invisible individuals. Teaching frankly about diverse identities can benefit everyone, as participants may have concerns or fears about their feelings and perceptions of their gender and/or sexual orientation.

9 SEX INVOLVES MORE THAN SEXUAL INTERCOURSE. Acknowledging this concept reminds participants that not only are there many ways to be sexual with a partner besides vaginal, oral and anal intercourse, but also that most of these other behaviors are safer and healthier than sexual intercourse.

CREATING A SUPPORTIVE ENVIRONMENT FOR LEARNING ABOUT SEXUAL HEALTH

A supportive group atmosphere and a supportive nonjudgmental educator are essential for sexual health education. Participants may be nervous, cautious, even suspicious as they address this sensitive issue, which requires a serious examination of their own behaviors. Since much of the learning occurs during interactions between group members, educators need to be effective group facilitators, creating a safe, nonthreatening environment in which people can talk openly and honestly about sexuality. The goal is to provide experiences that strengthen people's motivation and ability to take responsibility for their own sexual safety. A few basic interaction guidelines for educators include:

1. Establish "ground rules."

It is important that the educator help the group establish, and adhere to, clear guidelines for how the group will work together, so that everyone will feel safe and comfortable. If time allows, the educator can encourage participants to brainstorm their own ideas, with questions such as "What rules would you like to establish …?" and "What should we expect from everyone …?" The educator follows up with clarifying questions to help participants elaborate the ideas and take ownership of their ground rules. In a short session, the educator can post several of the most relevant time-honored ground rules (below), and ask for the group's agreement in carrying them out.

Key ground rules:
- Listen carefully.
- Respect people's right to express their own opinions, even if you disagree.
- Speak for yourself, not for others. Use "I" statements.
- Respect each other's confidentiality and privacy. Keep personal information in the group. (Rarely, an educator may need to break this rule if required by law or special circumstances.)
- Questions are welcome. There is no such thing as a "stupid" question.
- Every person has the right to pass on any activity or discussion.
- One person talks at a time. Avoid side conversations.
- Keep electronic devices turned off (and away).
- Think before you speak.
- No put downs. (No hurtful comments, looks, groans or gestures that would make anyone feel embarrassed, stupid or incompetent.)
- Share the time.
- Have fun!

Ground rules are sometimes called "group agreements" when working with adults. Here are some additional ideas for older groups:

- Assume good will.
- Listen to hear *and* understand ... not just respond.
- Limit side conversations.
- Speak from one's own experience.
- Use time thoughtfully and engage in your own way.
- Set your own boundaries for personal sharing.
- Use the language you currently have.
- Recognize participants are all in different places (personally and professionally).

Notes:

Ideas adapted with permission from many experienced educators and trainers, including Nora Gelperin, Maureen Kelly and Melissa Keyes DiGioia, and from Hedgepeth and Helmich.[*]

2. Use a Question Box.

Anonymous questions protect privacy and avoid embarrassment. A Question Box in a known but private place allows participants to submit concerns privately. Educators can also distribute small index cards and pencils, assuring anonymity, and ask everyone to write, even if it's only, "I do not have a question at this time." Educators may then approach each person to put questions in without anyone seeing what's on the cards. There is seldom a lack of questions in the box when a group is encouraged to learn about sexuality in this way. It's a good idea to wait a day before answering questions.

3. Encourage comfort and communication.

To the extent that it is in your control, try to ensure that the room is private and comfortable. Discourage interruptions that may distract and/or violate privacy. If possible, arrange chairs or desks in a circle or semi-circle so that participants can look at each other while talking. Balance the tone of the discussion so it is open, but not inappropriately personal for either the educator or the participants. Interactions that are humorous but not silly, fun but serious, can increase comfortable communication.

4. Use language that is inclusive and clear.

It is important to use inclusive, gender-neutral terms that do not assume everyone's gender identity or sexual orientation. This manual uses the pronouns "they," "them," and "their," rather than "she,"

---

[*] Hedgepeth, E., & Helmich, J. (1996). *Teaching about sexuality and HIV: Principles and methods for effective education*. New York: New York University Press.

"he," "her," and "his," wherever gender is not established. Other examples of inclusivity include statements such as, "A guy and his **partner** went to a party," rather than "a man and his **girlfriend** ...," or "What if a woman were going out with **someone** who wouldn't use protection?" rather than "with a **man** who wouldn't use protection?" or "What if a **man** refused to get tested at the same time as his partner?" are important for everyone to hear. Lesbian, gay, bisexual and transgender students will recognize the difference, which will make them feel safer and welcome.

Clarity is also important. Participants need to hear language they can understand. Sometimes using slang can be a very effective way to clarify information, as in "after the male **ejaculates, or 'cums.'"** It can be helpful to use sexual vernacular that is common among your participants. Phrases such as *hooking up* and *having sex* may assist you in meeting participants where they are. However, be aware that such language is often vague, and will need follow up clarification, e.g., "What do you think is meant by *hooking up*?"

5. Help participants think for themselves.

Education is supposed to help people **think,** not tell them what to do. The strategies in these lessons are designed to help people examine their own knowledge, attitudes, values and behaviors. Ideally, every response will demonstrate the educator's respect for the participant's potential to make healthy sexual decisions and build the self-efficacy needed to protect their sexual health. For educators to moralize or attempt to impose their own values is counterproductive. Here are some open-ended questions educators might ask:

- What do you think?
- What are the alternatives?
- What might/will happen if ...?
- What are the advantages? The disadvantages?
- What would you do?

6. Seek additional training in group facilitation.

It is important that educators who plan to teach about sexual health prepare themselves, especially if the above are new techniques for them. Professional development workshops can help them acquire the knowledge, attitudes and group facilitation skills needed to teach effectively. The American Association of Sexuality Educators, Counselors and Therapists lists upcoming trainings on their website, www.aasect.org. And each year, the CSE hosts a National Sex Ed Conference (see www.SexEdConference.com). Further, since sexual health information and recommendations may change, it is important for educators to keep themselves updated with respect to current data and resources.

HOW TO USE *SEX ED IN THE DIGITAL AGE*

Scope of the Manual

The lessons in this manual are **non-sequential** so educators can select those most relevant to their participants. It is important to know that *Sex Ed in the Digital Age* is **not a curriculum** and is not intended to be taught from start to finish. This resource focuses on the comfort, knowledge, attitudes and skills required for people to make responsible decisions about their sexual health. These materials can be used to *supplement* existing curricula in traditional academic or interdisciplinary settings, and the objectives and educational activities can be integrated into a variety of community settings.

How the Manual is Organized

Each lesson is designed to take approximately 45 minutes to one hour to complete, but the actual time needed will depend on the group, on participants' prior knowledge and experience, and on the importance the educator wants to give the topic. A few of these lessons can be completed in less time, but with more thorough discussion, many may take longer. Each lesson includes:

Objectives: The major learning participants will acquire from the lesson, in measurable terms.

Rationale: A brief explanation of the importance of that particular lesson.

Materials: Items needed for the lesson, plus related handouts and educator resources.

Procedure: A step-by-step guide to teaching the lesson.

A Resources Section at the end of the manual includes a description of different types of technology including apps and clickers, as well as social media platforms including Facebook, Instagram, Snapchat, Tumblr and Twitter.

Selection of Lessons and Activities

Few educators will use **all** of these lessons. However, in order to understand the scope of sex education, it is recommended that all educators read through the entire manual, particularly the rationales, to determine which lessons and activities will be most useful for the intended population.

As with all sex education materials, each activity needs to be carefully evaluated by the educator for its appropriateness in a particular community, with a particular group of participants at a particular time. Since these lessons are designed for use with a variety of ages, genders, backgrounds, etc., all activities will not be appropriate for all groups.

Permission

We are often asked about permission for reprinting the lessons that appear in our publications, and we are pleased to have granted permission to a number of leading health organizations throughout the world. Written permission from The Center for Sex Education is required for copying all material in *Sex Ed in the Digital Age*, with the exception of handouts, which may be freely copied in print format and distributed to participants in educational settings.

Written permission from The Center for Sex Education is required for reprinting other material (e.g., complete lessons, educator resources, etc.), or to post any material, including handouts, electronically. Please contact Info@SexEdCenter.org for further information.

HOW TO USE ROLE-PLAY

Rationale

Participants may know the "facts" about sexual health, safer sex and sexually transmitted infections, but unless they develop decision-making and communication skills for protecting themselves, they remain at high risk. Research suggests role-play is one of the most effective ways to develop the communication, negotiation and assertiveness skills essential for safer sex behaviors. Skill practice using role-play is an important part of any sexuality education effort, including the lessons in this manual, as it allows participants to apply what they have learned to real-life situations. If you ever have extra time in a given lesson, role-play is probably the best way to use it.

Benefits of Role-Play

Role-play helps participants:

1. Act out a wide variety of feelings and ideas without fear of judgment from others. Since they are "only acting," they can express and experience feelings and ideas that they often hide.

2. Try communicating ideas they may be reluctant to express in real life due to lack of confidence or knowledge, or to peer pressure.

3. Practice making decisions and identifying forces that influence decision making.

4. Evaluate how they solve problems and deal with the consequences of their behaviors.

5. Increase their problem-solving capabilities by generating alternatives.

6. Develop understanding and empathy for people who may have different experiences and opinions by acting as another person might in a particular situation.

7. Rehearse communication and assertiveness skills.

Before the Role-Play

1. Prepare yourself to facilitate the role-play. Think about your goals and decide how to organize the role-play to achieve those goals.

2. Be aware that role-play may trigger strong reactions in an individual who may suddenly realize that the situation or problem in some way applies to her/him. Consider how you will handle this without drawing undue attention to the participant; know what backup support you can call on for the person.

3. Prepare materials you need for the strategy you plan to use. "Character cards" describing each character are useful for getting started and large "character name tags" help participants stay in their roles and help the audience remember the "actors" are pretending to be someone else, not playing themselves.

4. Decide who needs to know what information about the role-play. What does the audience need to know about the situation? The characters? What do the characters need to know about each other? Are there any "secrets" that need to be maintained for the role-play to be effective?

5. If you have access to recording equipment, consider recording the role-play. Evaluate the pros and cons. Participants often like to see and hear themselves "on stage." They can examine their role-playing and get feedback from their peers. Consider how your group will benefit. Will role-play build or decrease participants' confidence? Can you arrange for smooth, trouble-free use of the equipment? If you do record the role-play, be sure that you, not participants, are fully in charge of the recording so it doesn't wind up on YouTube!

Simple Role-Play Strategies

Role-plays can be structured in a variety of ways, depending on the educator's skill and the group's level of functioning and willingness to participate. *However,* participants may have difficulty improvising at first. Using these *simple* strategies first can provide an opportunity for a person to develop communication skills in ways that are nonthreatening for both educators and participants. Establish ground rules that assure all group members will feel safe. Affirm and support participants as they develop these skills.

1. Ask two or three volunteers to act out a few written, realistic dialogues.

2. Ask pairs of volunteers to read or act out written realistic dialogues.

3. Give the participants several written "pressure lines" (e.g., "You would if you loved me …") and ask them in pairs to write one-line responses. Ask participants to read ("role-play") responses back to you.

4. Have participants do the same as #3 above, but with pairs writing and role-playing their own responses.

5. Create a dialogue with the group. Give them the first line and ask them to suggest how each person could respond in turn. Write the dialogue on a board/flip chart paper. Then ask a volunteer to act it out with you.

6. Create another dialogue with the group. Ask two volunteers to read it aloud.

7. Divide participants into pairs. Distribute a magazine picture of a couple to each pair. Ask pairs to write the opening lines in an imaginary dialogue the couple could have as they begin a discussion about safer sex. Encourage pairs to develop an exchange of at least four statements and

responses. Ask each pair to stand, one at a time, hold up their picture, and speak their dialogue to each other.

8. Divide participants into small groups and give each group a card describing a problem situation. Each group discusses its problem and possible strategies to deal with it. Next tell the group to select one of the strategies and write out a short role-play which they will then present to the entire group.

Steps to Effective Improvisational Role-Plays

1. **Set ground rules.** Explain that role-play is a great way to think about situations people may experience sometime in real life and to practice handling tough problems. Tell participants the success of any role-play depends upon how well they follow the five simple ground rules below:

   a. People playing roles need to **act** and **think** like the character would in the given situation. Observers need to be quiet and attentive, unless they are assigned another task.

   b. Role-players should say what comes to mind, not think too much before speaking.

   c. No one should "put down" the role-players, or anyone else in the room. (Emphasize this rule.)

   d. Respect privacy and confidentiality. (Whatever a person has said, either inside or outside the group, is not identified by that person's name; no asking of personal questions is appropriate; speak for one's self only.)

   e. Have fun, but stay focused.

2. **Organize the room comfortably.** Depending on the type of role-play you have chosen, consider setting up chairs at the front of the room, since participants usually feel more comfortable sitting than standing, at least at first. Make sure those observing can see and hear well.

3. **Identify the players.** You may ask for "impromptu" volunteers or ask someone to take on a role beforehand. No one should be forced to role-play, but often a little encouragement in advance works wonders. Pass out character cards or character name tags if needed.

4. **Set the scene.** Describe the situation. Make the issues between the characters clear. Then, draw a verbal picture of the location: "It's raining outside. You are sitting in the living room in front of the TV. Your mom is upstairs and … "

5. **Help characters get into their roles.** Ask one or two questions that will help each player begin to talk as the character might, and think about how that person is feeling. For example, "Derek, tell me about yourself." "How do you get along with your parents?" "What's the problem you're having with your sister?" Spend at most a minute with each character.

6. **Get the role-players started.** Explain exactly where the situation is at this moment. "So, you've been discussing this issue and you're both getting really angry. It's all yours now, you two!"

7. **Pay attention to the audience as well as the role-players.** If someone seems to be getting upset (flushed, agitated, tearful, head down on desk), handle it in a way that protects and respects their privacy and works in your setting.

8. **If necessary, refocus the role-play.** If the role-players are struggling so much that nothing is being accomplished, stop the role-play for a moment. Acknowledge that sometimes role-play (or that particular situation) may be difficult to enact. Make a suggestion to the players or ask observers for a suggestion. Or, ask if a player would like to have someone else try one of the roles, and handle accordingly.

9. **Stop the role-play.** When the problem is resolved or when it seems a good time to discuss the scene, stop the role-play. Remember that debriefing and a follow-up discussion are **vital** parts of role-play, so be sure to allow sufficient time for them.

10. **Have the audience ask questions of the players with the players *remaining in character*.** Questions and comments from the audience will help everyone examine the behaviors and alternatives that might have been possible in the situation. Comments and questions should focus on what the players did as the characters, ***not*** on how well they acted.

11. **Debrief the players.** Ask the players how they felt as their character in the role-play. What did they like or dislike about how they handled the problem? If the necessary trust level has developed in the group, ask how similar this situation is to those they have seen in real life. (Stress that no names should be mentioned.)

12. **Discuss the role-play.** The purpose of this discussion is to examine how the characters felt and behaved. It is ***not*** to evaluate the acting ability of the players. Discussion questions might include:

    a. What feelings do you have about any of the characters?

    b. What could any of the characters have done to improve the outcome of the situation?

    c. How do you think _____ felt when _____ (such a thing happened)?

    d. What do you admire about any of the characters?

    e. How difficult would this situation be to resolve in real life? Explain.

    f. What did you learn from observing this role-play?

Ideas for More Complex Improvisational Role-Plays

1. **Use *doubles*.** Have a second participant stand behind each player and occasionally suggest an idea to the player. The player may choose to use or not use the suggestion.

2. **Have role-players begin to act out a scenario.** At the point of highest tension, stop the action by saying, "***Freeze!***" Ask the audience how they think each of the characters is feeling. Ask for suggestions for resolving the conflict. Now have the role-players continue the role-play using one or more of those suggestions.

3. **Reverse *roles*.** At some point during the role-play, have players switch roles. For example, ask the female to become the male or the passive partner the assertive one, and vice versa. Restart the role-play.

4. **Use groups of three or four who will independently and simultaneously act out a situation.** Include an observer, and give participants points to be looking for in the interaction, as well as guidelines for their small-group discussion afterward. Allow enough time for enough role-plays so that each participant has the chance to play more than one role, including that of the observer.

5. **Use group-assisted and supported role-play.** It's useful to make character cards (large index cards to which information about one character is affixed) and character name tags (hung around character's neck during role-play).

   Note:
   Punch two holes at the top of each card. Cut about three feet of yarn for each card, pull the yarn through the holes and knot at both ends to create a name tag that fits loosely around the neck. (See example.)

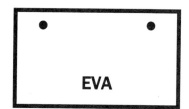

   a. Divide participants into small groups, explaining that each group will focus on one character in the role-play scenario. Give each group one of the role-play character cards and each individual a small index card. The group is to read the description and discuss how its character will act in the role-play. After about five minutes, ask the group to select one volunteer to take part in the role-play.

   b. Tell the other group members that, as the role-play progresses, they are to write on their cards any suggestions they have for the actor from their group about what else he/she might do or say. At specified times they will be able to deliver these suggestions to their actor, who may choose to use the suggestions or ignore them.

   c. Ask the actors to come forward. Help them get into their roles by asking, "How are you feeling about the situation right now?" Tell the players to begin the scene. Let the role-play continue as long as it seems productive, but no more than 10 minutes.

d. Now ask the actors to return to their own groups to get more suggestions. A new person may assume the role at this time. Have the actors begin again, continuing the role-play. (Group members may also continue to make written suggestions to their actor.)

e. Stop the role-play in time to debrief the actors and help them get out of their roles. Ask each, "How did you feel in the role that you played?"

Discussion Questions:

a. What examples can you give of something a character did or said that *encouraged* communication? Something that *discouraged* communication?

b. Why might the characters not have talked about this situation sooner?

c. What would you recommend to the characters about future discussions of this situation?

CONTENTS

By Carolyn Cooperman, MA, MSW
In this lesson, participants will use their online skills to relate to the ways in which life improves when rights that were once denied are ultimately granted. Participants begin to understand that as in all human rights struggles, progress is made through activism, legislation and support from the broader population.

Looking at Gender, Sexual Orientation, Risk and More
By Carolyn Cooperman, MA, MSW
It is important that teens have some criteria to use when navigating the social landscape and forming relationships online. This lesson will allow all participants to explore the topic of e-flirting personally, without the predominant emphasis placed on heterosexual flirting.

Promoting an Inclusive School Environment for LGBTQ Youth through Project-Based Learning
By Hannah M. Priest, CHES, MAED, Christine L. Hackman, MA and Sarah E. Rush, MA
Project-based learning is a student-centered instructional technique that requires students to think critically, problem solve and collaborate. By utilizing accessible technology, students will work in groups to develop and implement a creative strategy that will be used to promote an inclusive school environment for LGBTQ students.

Section 4
Creating Safe, Inclusive Programs

No single norm fits all teenagers. We have arrived at an age when bullying teenagers for differences in physical appearance, gender, sexual orientation, sexual behavior, etc. is unacceptable. Anti-bullying campaigns are certainly important; however they alone will not eradicate intolerant behavior. The culture at large has to change. The lessons in this section, as well as in others included elsewhere in these volumes, begin with the assumption that the participants in each and every group will be sexually and developmentally diverse. The lessons strive to recognize, normalize and acknowledge the needs of all of the potential participants. Lessons in this section include:

Googling Human Rights

E-Flirting:
Looking at Gender, Sexual Orientation, Risk and More

Engaging Generation Z in Peer-Driven Advocacy:
Promoting an Inclusive School Environment for LGBTQ
Youth through Project-Based Learning

Rallying against Bullying

GOOGLING HUMAN RIGHTS

By Carolyn Cooperman, MA, MSW

Objectives

By the end of this lesson, participants will be able to:

1. Use Internet skills to research U.S. human rights legislation that has improved the quality of life for participants and their families.

2. Assess the current status of the LGBTQ (lesbian, gay, bisexual, transgender and questioning) human rights movement in the United States.

3. Explain how human rights evolve as a result of activism, legislation and support from the population at large.

Rationale

The struggle to advance human rights in this country began with the drafting of the U.S. Constitution and continues to this day. Along with the many freedoms that Americans now enjoy, the challenge to eliminate inequity and discrimination is ongoing. In this lesson, the effort to enact LGBTQ anti-discrimination legislation is studied as being one of the many battles that historically have been waged to expand human rights.

Young people use search engines to research information on the Internet so often that *Google* has become its own verb. In this lesson, they will use their online skills to relate to the ways in which life improves when rights that were once denied are ultimately granted. Participants begin to understand that as in all human rights struggles, progress is made through activism, legislation and support from the broader population.

Materials

- Flip chart paper or board, markers
- Computers, smartphones or tablets for conducting Internet research
- **Handout: Know Your Rights**
- **Educator Resource: Human Rights Questions and Answers**

Procedure

1. Ask participants, "What was the last thing you Googled?" Allow a few volunteers to respond.

Discussion Questions:

    a. What are some of the things that can be researched online?

    b. How do you research something online? What are the steps you take?

    c. How do you know the right words to search?

    d. How do you select a reliable source if you get too many results?

    e. How would you go about researching human rights issues online?

2. Explain that this lesson traces the progress of human rights achievements in the United States. Warm up by asking the following question: "Do you know what rights are granted in the U.S. Constitution under the First Amendment of the Bill of Rights?" Elicit responses and then call for a few volunteers to use electronic devices to search for information about First Amendment rights.

3. Write the following heading on the board/flip chart:

    The First Amendment of the Bill of Rights prevented the government from denying specific freedoms about:

    As the freedoms are read out loud by the volunteers, list them under the heading.

    Answers: religion, speech, the press, the right to peaceably assemble, the right to petition grievances

4. Ask the participants if the rights specified in the First Amendment were granted to all people who lived in the colonies at the time. The answer is no, only white males who owned land were granted First Amendment rights.

5. Draw a timeline on the board/flip chart. First Amendment rights were adopted into the Bill of Rights in 1791. Enter it onto the timeline.

    1700s   1800s   1900s   2000s

Discussion Questions:

    a. If First Amendment rights were only granted to white males who owned land, who was left out?

    b.   What are your feelings about people who were left out when it came to these rights?

    c.   In the United States, do you know of any other human rights that were fought for over time?

    d.   Why are First Amendment rights important?

6.   Distribute the **Handout: Know Your Rights** which traces landmark human rights decisions throughout U.S. history. Divide the participants into small groups. For expediency, **assign only one question on the handout to each group.** Direct the participants to find the answers online using a computer, smartphone or tablet. Additional questions can be assigned as time permits.

   For the correct answers, see the **Educator Resource: Human Rights Questions and Answers.**

7.   Allow 15 minutes for the participants to complete their research online. Reconvene, and review their findings. As each group reports, enter their findings onto the timeline.

   Discussion Questions:

    a.   Which of the human rights issues that we talked about today were at one time denied to your great-grandparents, grandparents or parents? Are any of your relatives still being denied basic human rights, in the United States or elsewhere?

    b.   How do human rights laws eventually get enacted?

    c.   Which human rights issues remain controversial, even though laws have been enacted?

    d.   Why do you think it takes so long to enact human rights legislation?

    e.   What does it mean to be "on the right side of history"?

    f.   Which human rights laws are most important to you?

Know Your Rights

Directions: You will be assigned one item from the following list to research on the Internet. Keep your answers brief, but accurate. Write your answers on a separate piece of paper.

1. What legislation eventually abolished slavery in the United States and when was it enacted?

2. What U.S. legislation granted women the right to vote and when was it enacted?

3. What was the Civil Rights Movement in the United States?

4. What is the Civil Rights Act of 1964?

5. What is the Equal Pay Act of 1963 and what did it specify? Do women now earn equal pay for equal work?

6. What is *Roe v. Wade,* when was it decided by the Supreme Court, and what right does it protect?

7. What were the Stonewall Riots and when did they occur?

8. What is "Don't Ask, Don't Tell," and is this policy still in effect in the United States today?

9. What is *United States v. Windsor,* when was it decided, and what rights does it grant to same-sex couples who are married?

10. The DREAM Act (Development, Relief, and Education for Alien Minors Act) is pending legislation that was first introduced in the Senate in 2001, but has not yet been passed in both houses of Congress. It proposes a plan for allowing minors who entered the United States illegally, yet have lived and gone to school here, to work towards permanent residency. What proposed standards do the minors who entered this country illegally have to meet in order to eventually be granted permanent residency?

Human Rights Questions and Answers[1]

The questions and answers below correspond to the **Handout: Know Your Rights.**

1. **What legislation eventually abolished slavery in the United States and when was it enacted?**

   Most of the Northern colonies and territories began abolishing slavery after the Revolutionary War. They did not want the government to deny people of their basic right to be free. The Southern territories wanted slavery for economic reasons, primarily to supply labor for the cotton industry. It took the Civil War to reconcile the differences between North and South. The Emancipation Proclamation, an executive order signed by President Abraham Lincoln, abolished slavery in the Confederate States on January 1, 1863. **The Thirteenth Amendment** to the Constitution permanently outlawed slavery throughout all the United States, except as punishment for a crime. The Thirteenth Amendment was officially adopted on **December 6, 1865.**

2. **What U.S. legislation granted women the right to vote and when was it enacted?**

   Women's suffrage, or the right to vote, was achieved over time through group organization, rallies and protests. Some states advanced suffrage before the federal government made strides in granting women the right to vote, but **in 1920, the Nineteenth Amendment to the Constitution** was passed. This Amendment proclaims: "the right of citizens of the United States to vote shall not be denied or abridged by the United States or by any State on account of sex."

3. **What was the Civil Rights Movement in the United States?**

   The slow progress in ending racial discrimination gave rise to the Civil Rights Movement (roughly 1954-1968). Marches, sit-ins, protests and other acts of civil disobedience were primarily used to draw attention to and eliminate segregation in schools, restaurants, public transportation, etc. These efforts not only worked to improve anti-discrimination legislation, but also worked to change attitudes about segregation in the population at large.

4. **What is the Civil Rights Act of 1964?**

   The Civil Rights Act of 1964 was an outgrowth of the Civil Rights Movement. It outlawed major forms of discrimination against African-Americans and women. It is a federal law ending unequal

---

[1] Unless otherwise noted, the material in this handout comes from www.Wikipedia.org.

voter registration requirements and segregation in the workplace and other facilities that served the general public. The Civil Rights Act of 1964 was signed into law by President Lyndon B. Johnson.

5. **What is the Equal Pay Act of 1963 and what did it specify? Do women now earn equal pay for equal work?**

The Equal Pay Act of 1963 is **a federal law aimed at abolishing wage discrimination based on gender.** It was signed into law by John F. Kennedy and it **prevents employers from paying lower wages to employees of one gender over another.** When employees perform equal work on jobs requiring equal skill and responsibilities, and work under similar working conditions, they deserve equal pay. To date however, women still earn 77 cents for every dollar earned by men.[2]

6. **What is *Roe v. Wade,* when was it decided by the Supreme Court, and what right does it protect?**

Roe v. Wade was a 1973 Supreme Court decision that legalized abortion in the United States. A woman's right to a safe, legal abortion could not be denied by state or federal laws. A woman's right to privacy, protected by a clause under the Fourteenth Amendment, meant that the choice to have an abortion was to be made by a woman and her doctor, not the government. *Roe v. Wade* was an outgrowth of the Women's Liberation Movement. Reproductive freedoms were among the many freedoms that women were advocating for during the 1960s and 1970s. This ruling proved to be extremely polarizing, with groups for and against abortion rights vehemently advocating for their respective positions.

7. **What were the Stonewall Riots and when did they occur?**

The Stonewall riots consisted of violent demonstrations by members of the gay community against a police raid of the Stonewall Inn, located in Greenwich Village, in New York City. The Stonewall riots are considered by many to be the most influential event that gave rise to the gay liberation movement, and the modern fight for gay and lesbian rights in the United States.

8. **What is "Don't Ask, Don't Tell," and is this policy still in effect in the United States today?**

"Don't Ask, Don't Tell' was an official U.S. policy about homosexuals serving in the military. Military personnel were prohibited from asking questions about a person's sexual orientation and service members were required to conceal information about their sexual orientation. Those who

---

[2] The White House. (n.d.). Did you know that women are still paid less than men? Retrieved July 18, 2014 from www.whitehouse.gov/equal-pay/career

were outspoken faced possible discharge from the service. This policy was officially repealed on September 20, 2011 after the Secretary of Defense, the Joint Chiefs of Staff, and President Barack Obama all agreed that lesbian and gay people posed no threat to combat readiness or national security. People of all sexual orientations can now serve openly in the armed services, officially free from discrimination or harassment.

9. **What is *United States v. Windsor,* when was it decided, and how does it affect same-sex couples who are married?**

United States v. Windsor is a decision handed down by the U.S. Supreme Court on June 26, 2013. The ruling held Section 3 of the Defense of Marriage Act to be unconstitutional. Now, same-sex couples that are married can receive the same *federal* marriage benefits that those in traditional marriages are allowed, such as filing joint tax returns, exemption from estate taxes, and making end of life decisions. This ruling does not legalize same-sex marriage in all fifty states. At the time of this printing, individual states must pass their own legislation to allow same-sex marriage. Check to see if same-sex marriage is allowed in your state.

10. **The DREAM Act (Development, Relief, and Education for Alien Minors Act) is pending legislation that was first introduced in the Senate in 2001, but has not yet been passed in both houses of Congress. It proposes a plan for allowing minors who entered the United States illegally, yet have lived and gone to school here, to work towards permanent residency. What proposed standards do the minors who entered this country illegally have to meet in order to eventually be granted permanent residency?**

To be granted permanent residency, they have to be of good moral character, and have either acquired a degree from an institution of higher education in the United States or have completed at least two years in good standing in a program for a bachelor's or higher degree in the United States. Service in the armed services for at least two years, with an honorable discharge, is another way of working towards permanent residency.

At the time of this printing, Congress has not passed immigration reform legislation. There is considerable pressure from the Latino community and other human rights advocacy groups to provide funds for college tuition for illegal residents to help them move ahead. Additionally, specific guidelines are needed for a more humane pathway to citizenship. This issue will continue to be kept in the forefront until legislation is passed.

E-FLIRTING
Looking at Gender, Sexual Orientation, Risk and More

By Carolyn Cooperman, MA, MSW

Objectives

By the end of this lesson, participants will be able to:

1. Understand why and how people flirt, regardless of gender or sexual orientation.

2. Create simulated text exchanges that involve thinking about how to initiate or respond to flirtatious communications.

3. Evaluate some of the stereotypes about gender and sexual orientation with regard to flirting.

Rationale

In schoolyards, lunchrooms and classrooms, flirtatious behavior is easy to spot. Electronic flirting, however, among those who are either known to one another or becoming acquainted for the first time, travels below the radar. With the advent of texting, email and social networking sites, the social field has expanded far beyond the school community. For this reason, it becomes particularly important that teens have some criteria to use when navigating the social landscape and forming relationships online.

Female, male, heterosexual and LGBTQ (lesbian, gay, bisexual, transgender and questioning) participants can take part in this lesson from their own vantage points. All can explore the topic personally, without the predominant emphasis placed on heterosexual flirting. The best sexuality education programs take an integrated approach, considering how all can benefit from the topic under consideration. LGBT participants, who in general are not as free to flirt openly, will undoubtedly be drawn to the anonymity of electronic flirting. This makes it all the more necessary that everyone be included, in a natural and upfront manner, when exploring this topic.

Materials
- **Handout: Examples of Flirting via Text Messages**

Procedure
1. Explain that the lesson is going to be about flirting via text messages. Begin by providing a working definition of the term *flirting.* This sets the tone for how the term will be used throughout the lesson.

Definition: Flirting involves behavior that indicates an interest in another person, with or without a sexual intent. For example, it is believed that even babies engage in a distinct type of eye contact to establish a connection with a parent or caregiver. Flirting can range from simply liking someone else, to being indicative of a sexual attraction. While it is normal for people of all genders and sexual orientations to flirt, there are those who don't for a variety of reasons.

Discussion Questions:

a. What kind of person-to-person flirting is noticeable in school or other social settings? *(Point out that flirting can occur in a split second. Non-verbal signals — such as raised eyebrows, eye-contact, hair flick, playing with accessories, leaning in, sideway glances, laughter, etc. — are common signs of flirting).*

b. What kinds of flirting do you think are acceptable in public? Unacceptable? Explain.

c. What are some of the ways that people flirt online or through texts?

d. How does in-person flirting differ from electronic flirting?

2. Divide the group into pairs and distribute the **Handout: Examples of Flirting via Text Messages.** There are four scenarios on the handout. If time permits, the participants can address all four examples. If not, assign only one or two scenarios to each pair. Several pairs can work on the same example to elicit a variety of responses.

Allow time for the participants to complete the handout. Reconvene and review their responses.

Discussion Questions:

a. What was it like to give gender and sexual orientation assignments to the characters in your scenarios? How did you make this decision?

b. If you were to change these assignments, would the dialogue you created still work? Why, or why not? (Actually demonstrate this by taking one of the text exchanges and altering the gender and sexual orientation assignments.)

c. What stereotypes about gender and sexual orientation are noticeable when addressing the topic of flirting?

d. Does flirting just come naturally or do you have to give some thought to how to do this effectively?

e. What types of flirtatious texts are effective? Which are offensive?

f.   What's the difference between a real and a false sexual portrayal?

g.   How should a person respond to an unwanted sexual overture?

h.   Do you believe it is important for a person of sexual interest to know something about your interests, activities, personality, etc.? Why, or why not?

3.   Conclude by asking half of the participants to discuss, in pairs, one piece of advice they would give to a person who received UNWANTED flirting via text. The other participants should discuss, also in pairs, one piece of advice they would give to a person who received WANTED flirting via text.

4.   Ask for several participants to share their advice.

Examples of Flirting via Text Messages

Directions: Below are examples of different ways that people flirt via text messages. You will notice that in each example, there are no specific details given about the gender or the sexual orientation of the characters involved.

> **Step 1:** You are to decide the gender and sexual orientation of the characters in the scene. Give names to your characters.

> **Step 2**: In the space provided, simulate a text exchange between the characters. Pass the paper back and forth and add entries as if the characters were texting one another.

Example 1: A fifteen-year-old wants to text a person of interest. This person shares several of the same classes and they have known one another for a long time. This is the first time that the 15-year-old will act on a strong attraction via text messaging and there is uncertainty about how to do this effectively. Help this character get started, followed by a text exchange between the two.

Example 2: Two teenagers who are unknown to one another will be meeting for the first time via text messaging. They will introduce themselves to one another by providing some information about themselves. Friends thought they would like one another and set them up to meet. Decide how they will portray themselves to one another.

Example 3: A 17-year-old is very sexually attracted to a classmate and will let this be known to the person of interest via text messages. The text under consideration is not really true to the way that this person wants to act in a relationship, but thinks that this is what is expected in a sexual exchange. You decide whether the character will start a text exchange that is true to feelings or a false representation of sexual interest.

Example 4: A teenager has been receiving complimentary, flirtatious texts from a school coach. This has been going on for a while. You decide the way in which the coach flirts and how the recipient should respond.

ENGAGING GENERATION Z IN PEER-DRIVEN ADVOCACY:
Promoting an Inclusive School Environment for LGBTQ Youth through Project-Based Learning

By Hannah M. Priest, CHES, MAED, Christine L. Hackman, MA and Sarah E. Rush, MA[*]

Objectives

By the end of this lesson, participants will be able to:

1. Explain why advocating for an inclusive school environment for students who identify as LGBTQ (lesbian, gay, bisexual, transgender or questioning) is necessary and important.

2. Describe two or more technology-based strategies to promote an inclusive school environment for students who identify as LGBTQ.

3. Implement one innovative, technology-based strategy to promote an inclusive school environment for LGBTQ students.

Rationale

LGBTQ youth face substantial adversity in today's society, one which favors heterosexuality, demonizes other sexual identities and forms of sexual expression, and shames gender non-confirming characteristics.[1] Identifying as LGBT is associated with a higher risk of harassment and discrimination victimization, which can lead to unhealthy coping and the pursuit of risky behaviors. A healthy school environment intentionally promotes an inclusive and positive emotional climate where students feel accepted, supported and involved, regardless of differences. A recent national study found that students involved in an intentionally inclusive environment were more likely to report that they felt more connected to their student community and that their peers were somewhat or very accepting of LGBT individuals.[2]

---

[*] Hannah M. Priest, CHES, MAED, Christine L. Hackman, MA and Sarah E. Rush, MA, are Health Education and Promotion doctoral students at The University of Alabama, Tuscaloosa.

[1] Advocates for Youth. (2008). Gay, lesbian, bisexual, transender and questioning (GLBTQ) youth. Retrieved July 19, 2014 from http://www.advocatesforyouth.org/publications/424

[2] Kosciw, J. G., Greytak, E. A., Bartkiewicz, M. J., Boesen, M. J., & Palmer, N. A. (2012). *The 2011 National School Climate Survey: The experiences of lesbian, gay, bisexual and transgender youth in our nation's schools*. New York: Gay, Lesbian & Straight Education Network (GLSEN).

Project-based learning is a student-centered instructional technique that requires students to think critically, problem solve and collaborate. This technique involves opportunities for revision and deeper reflection on the topic. By utilizing accessible technology, students will work in groups to develop and implement a creative strategy that will be used to promote an inclusive school environment for LGBTQ students.

Materials

- Flip chart paper or board, markers
- Computers, tablets or smartphones with Internet access
- **Handout: Advocating for an Inclusive School Environment via Technology**.

Note:

Prior to this lesson, participants should be able to differentiate gender identity and sexual orientation. Participants should also know the **LGBTQ** acronym. If not, this should be addressed at the beginning of the lesson.

Procedure

1. To begin the session, draw a circle on the board/flip chart and write **DISCRIMINATION FACED BY LGBTQ YOUTH IN SCHOOLS** in the center of the circle. Ask participants to share responses to the following question: **What are some examples of discrimination that LGBTQ students may face at school?** Draw straight lines from the circle to record participants' responses at the ends of these lines.

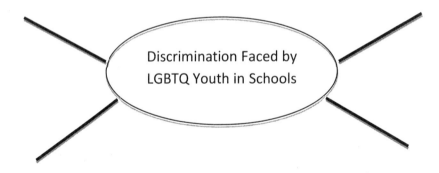

2. Once all of the participant responses are recorded, ask the following questions.

   Discussion Questions:

   a. How do you think discrimination affects LGBTQ students?

   b. Why is it important to promote an inclusive school environment for LGBTQ students?

   c. What can be done to prevent LGBTQ discrimination from occurring in schools and/or in the community?

      d. What can you do *personally* to discourage LGBTQ discrimination in your own peer group? Give an example.

      e. How can you best spread the message of an inclusive school environment for students?

3. Tell participants, "So we see that LGBTQ students may face intentional exclusion or isolation from peers, verbal or physical harassment, and even physical assault. Consequently, LGBTQ students often engage in risky behaviors to help cope with discrimination and harassment. Today, you will have the opportunity to take steps to advocate for LGBTQ students and promote an inclusive school environment."

4. Ask participants to divide into small groups of approximately four to five individuals. Next, post the following question on the board/flip chart: **How can we use technology to best promote an inclusive school for LGBTQ students?**

5. Explain that each group will develop two innovative technology-based strategies to promote an inclusive school environment for LGBTQ students, and each group will implement one of their strategies. Emphasize the importance of practicality, especially for implementation purposes.

6. Provide students with the **Handout: Advocating for an Inclusive School Environment via Technology.** Allow participants to choose from the list and work with their groups to come up with two primary ideas.

7. As groups work together, walk around and answer any questions participants may have about the task. Provide each group with specific, verbal feedback about their ideas, and help them choose one primary strategy to develop and implement.

8. Each group develops and implements their facilitator-approved strategy. If time allows, each group can share their advocacy efforts with other groups.

9. Debrief the participants with the following questions.

    Discussion Questions:

      a. As we discussed earlier, creating an inclusive school environment for LGBTQ students is a crucial task. What is the most important thing you learned from this activity?

b. Promoting an inclusive school environment is not always an easy task. What is one of the challenges you and your group faced during this activity?

c. What are some other ways you can promote an inclusive school environment for LGBTQ students in your daily life?

10. Conclude by explaining to participants that there are various methods to promote inclusivity for LGBTQ students within the school environment, and encourage them to continue brainstorming new methods to do so for the future.

Advocating for an Inclusive School Environment via Technology

Directions:

1. First, consider the following question with your group members: **How can we use technology to best promote an inclusive school for LGBTQ students?**

2. As a group, choose two of the media below that you can use to demonstrate advocacy and promote an inclusive school environment for LGBTQ students. You may also use other media, but check to ensure that they are appropriate for the task.

3. Brainstorm two strategies to promote an inclusive school environment for LGBTQ students.

4. Work with the educator to determine which strategy may be most effective with an audience and also realistic to implement.

5. Once consensus has been reached, work with your group to develop an advocacy message, and implement the strategy. You will share your work with other groups.

6. Keep in mind that you want to target as many people as possible, and also use a method that is user friendly, and may be easily replicated by others.

Medium options

- Information graphic development and dissemination (www.infogr.am)
- Vine (free app available at www.vine.co)
- Keek (short video clip uploads at www.keek.com)
- Edublogs (available at www.edublogs.org)
- Social media sites:
    - Facebook (www.facebook.com)
    - Instagram (www.instagram.com)
    - Twitter (www.twitter.com)
- Google+ (https://plus.google.com/)
- Others apps that are free, practical, and relevant (must be facilitator-approved)

Resource to help

- GLSEN's *Safe Space Kit: Guide to Being an Ally to LGBT Students.* Available for purchase or download at http://glsen.org/safespace.

Strategy 1

Medium:

Message:

How will you implement it?

Strategy 2

Medium:

Message:

How will you implement it?

RALLYING AGAINST BULLYING

By Carolyn Cooperman, MA, MSW

Objectives

By the end of this lesson, participants will be able to:

1. Use their technological and artistic talents to demonstrate how teens can counter cyberbullying.

2. Identify specific strategies for intervening when others are being bullied.

3. Understand how to support the victims of cyberbullying.

Rationale

Among the teens who use social networking sites, 88% report that they have witnessed mean or cruel online communications.[1] To address teenage uncertainty about what to do when damaging texts, photos or postings circulate, this lesson challenges participants to use their skills in technology, music, art, writing, drama, etc. to lead a peer-initiated response to cyberbullying. Participants develop projects that demonstrate how prevention, intervention and support can all be employed to counter the damaging effects of online bullying. Sexual themes, such as LGBTQ (lesbian, gay, bisexual, transgender and questioning) bullying, offensive gender stereotyping and the circulation of photos without consent, are included on the list of recommended projects. Ultimately, the projects participants design are reviewed by the group, with the intention of using them more broadly in school campaigns. The review process in itself is a means to both teach and inspire about counteracting cyberbullying.

Materials

- Flip chart paper or board, markers
- Electronic equipment (e.g., computers, Smart Board, amplifiers, copiers, etc.) that will enable participants to create and present their projects to the group
- **Handout: Peer Projects to Counter Cyberbullying**

Note:
This activity requires several weeks to complete.

---

[1] Pew Research Center. (November 9, 2011). Teens, kindness and cruelty on social network sites. Retrieved July 22, 2014 from http://pewInternet.org/Press-Releases/2011/Teens-and-social-media.aspx

Procedure

1. Begin by asking: "How many of you have seen someone being mean or cruel to another person on a social networking site? What are some of the things that people can do when they see bullying or harassing on texts, pictures and social networking sites?" Allow several volunteers to comment.

   Write the following on the board/flip chart:

   <u>**What Every Teen Can Do To Help**</u>
   Prevention
   Intervention
   Support

2. Explore the above categories by asking participants to explain how the terms relate to cyberbullying.

   Prevention *is a means for stopping bullying and harassment before it starts, primarily by raising public awareness through announcements, songs, posters, etc.*

   Intervention *requires actions that interrupt bullying and harassment while in progress.*

   Support *offers help and assistance to those who have already been bullied or harassed.*

   Examples that illustrate each of these terms can be found in the **Handout: Peer Projects to Counter Cyberbullying.**

3. Distribute the **Handout: Peer Projects to Counter Cyberbullying,** which outlines an assignment and provides ideas for selecting and designing a project. Review and clarify the handout so that everyone is clear about what the assignment entails.

4. All projects must be approved prior to implementation. Provide the participants with the required completion date.

   Post signs (**Prevention, Intervention, Support**) around the room and direct the students to stand by the category that interests them most. If any of the groups are too large, break them down by counting off, or by any fair way the group leader devises (in a lesson on bullying, no participant should feel excluded).

5. Over the next few sessions, monitor how the projects are progressing.

6. Assess the amount of session time needed to view all of the presentations. Have the participants make their presentations, followed by the selection of one or two projects that excelled in originality and effectiveness. End by acknowledging all of the contributions made by the participants.

   Discussion Questions:

   a. Would you like to see any of these projects implemented in this school?

   b. Did you get any good ideas about how you might intervene if a friend was being bullied?

   c. How is cyber bullying similar to in-person bullying? How is it different?

   d. Do any of these projects interest you personally?

   e. What do you think teens can do to stop cyber bullying that parents and teachers might not be able to accomplish?

7. Projects being considered for use in school-wide campaigns should be passed along to the school administration for approval.

Peer Projects to Counter Cyberbullying

Use your skills in graphic art, music, video production, writing, drawing, acting, etc. to illustrate any of the ideas listed below. Feel free to develop an original idea of your own. All projects must be approved and ready to present to the group by _____. You may complete the projects in groups or work on your own.

IDEAS FOR PROJECTS

Prevention:

Use any clever, creative means that you can think of to:

- Discourage the sending of embarrassing pictures without consent.

- Discourage the spread of sexual rumors or lies.

- Discourage the bullying of LGBTQ students.

- Let people know that sexual insults are not OK.

- Portray the type of bullying that many girls want to stop.

- Portray the type of bullying that many boys want to stop.

- Illustrate how cyberbullying damages self-esteem.

Intervention:

- Develop a graphic that can be uploaded onto an electronic device and sent back to offenders upon the receipt of a bullying text or posting.

- Create a short written message that can be transmitted following an incident of online bullying.

- Find a way to show that a potential consequence of cyberbullying is being "defriended" on a social networking site.

- Invite an offender to join a club that plays constructive, non-violent video games as an alternative to bullying. Establish a plan for how to get such a group together, make suggestions for a variety of games that would be appealing to teens, etc., and develop a video to advertise your club.

- Create a Twitter handle that calls out bullying whenever it happens.

Support:

- Offer step-by-step guidelines for how to survive in school following an incident of cyberbullying. This could be in the form of a written manual or video that can be posted on the school website. Portray what to say to those who ridicule; how to walk down the halls confidently in the face of embarrassment, etc. This project is meant to promote confidence and bolster self-esteem.

- Video a group of teens who have been cyberbullied in different ways. Have them describe what is OK online, and what is not.

- Create a series of short videos (under 15-30 seconds) that can be used to demonstrate assertive responses to cyberbullying.

- Create a comic book that illustrates how students can help out when friends are cyberbullied.

- Create a video that demonstrates how to report an incident of cyberbullying.

Section 5
Privacy, Consent and Safety

Adolescents have a difficult time understanding that text messages between friends do not necessarily remain private. Nor is it easy to comprehend the idea that simple messages sent via the Internet can potentially be seen by anyone, all over the world. The lessons in this section work to help teens employ self-protective measures for maintaining their own privacy, and to explore circumstances that might impinge upon the privacy of others. Internet safety, an issue of primary importance, involves utilizing criteria to assess potential risk factors when meeting unknown people online. Lessons in this section include:

If It's Private, Don't Post It!

You Can't Get It Back

Text Then Sext … What Happens Next

Think Before You Text

**Safer Cyber Sex:
Exploring Online Relationships**

IF IT'S PRIVATE, DON'T POST IT

By Carolyn Cooperman, MA, MSW

Objectives

By the end of this lesson, participants will be able to:

1. Analyze situations that demonstrate how private moments can become public when information is transmitted electronically.

2. Know the advantages and limitations of privacy settings on social networking sites.

3. Evaluate safety measures that protect privacy.

Rationale

If you have ever tried to set the privacy controls on a social networking site, you will not be surprised to learn that 66% of adult Facebook users reported that they did not know how to adjust the privacy controls.[1] How then can we expect the 73% of teens who are on a social network to be any better equipped to restrict wall posts to limited "friends," or to understand that much of what they believe to be private can easily be accessed by an audience much larger than their select friends?[2] This lesson demonstrates how well-intended measures to safeguard privacy can fail, resulting in potential embarrassment, harassment and review by colleges and future employers. The take-away message is clear: The safest way to protect private information is to refrain from posting it in the first place.

Materials

- Flip chart paper or board, markers
- **Handout: When Private Moments Become Public**
- **Handout: Tips for Staying Safe Online**

Procedure

1. Begin the lesson by writing the following heading on the board/flip chart:

    Ways to prevent private information from "going viral" over the Internet

---

[1] Consumer Reports. (June 2012). Facebook & your privacy: Who sees the data you share on the biggest social network? Retrieved July 22, 2014 from http://www.consumerreports.org/cro/magazine/2012/06/facebook-your-privacy/index.htm

[2] Lenhart, A., Purcell, K., Smith, A., & Zickuhr, K. (February 3, 2010). Social media and young adults. Retrieved July 22, 2014 from http://www.pewinternet.org/Reports/2010/Social-Media-and-Young-Adults.aspx

Participants are to list as many ideas as possible, such as setting safety controls on social networking sites, limiting access of information to specific friends, not posting private info, password protection, etc. Review their responses and process with the following questions:

Discussion Questions:

a. How many of you have set the safety controls on an account such as Facebook, Tumblr, etc.? Why did you do so?

b. How do safety controls on social networking sites protect privacy? Do the safety controls fully guarantee privacy? Why or why not?

c. Of the methods we listed for protecting privacy, which method do you think is the most effective?

Conclude by mentioning that you will return to the issue of safety controls later on in the lesson.

2. The next part of the lesson is a small group activity that utilizes the **Handout: When Private Moments Become Public.** Three examples that illustrate failures to protect privacy are outlined in the handout. If time allows, the small groups can address all three examples. Alternatively, the examples can be divided up, with only one example assigned to each small group.

3. Allow time for the small groups to complete the assignment. Reconvene and review their responses. Follow up with a discussion.

Discussion Questions:

a. Do colleges and employers have the right to review your social networking account? *Laws are currently being enacted that limit this right. It is now illegal in several states for employers to demand access to social media accounts.*

b. Legal considerations aside, what kind of photos might you post that you *would* want a school or college to see?

c. If people are kissing or making out at parties, how likely is it that pictures will be taken?

d. How did people in these examples try protect their privacy? What else could they have done?

e. What do you think about the motto **"If it's private, don't post it"**? Do you think you will use this advice? Why or why not?

Note:

Suggest that participants who want to learn how to install privacy controls should check their accounts for instructions and report back about their results. Participants might also volunteer to help others learn how to set the controls.

4. Distribute the **Handout: Tips for Staying Safe Online.** Divide the groups into pairs and ask the participants to check two safety measures they currently use, and star two recommendations they most want to remember. Review the handout, and follow up with a discussion.

    Discussion Questions:

    a. Which of the recommendations are new to you?

    b. Are there any recommendations that you agree with? Why?

    c. Are there any recommendations that you do not agree with? Why?

    d. Which recommendations are you currently using?

    e. Which recommendations do you most want to remember?

    f. Why should you use passwords and always lock down your devices?

    g. Have you heard about any other safety measures that people should know about?

When Private Moments Become Public

Directions: Read the following examples and answer the questions.

Example 1: A teenage girl took photos of her friends at a sleepover, posing in their underwear. She posted them on Facebook, feeling confident that the privacy controls on her account would limit circulation to select friends. Her father, who had access to her site but rarely screened her Facebook page, was alarmed to find the pictures in his newsfeed. He demanded that the pictures be deleted, took away her cellphone, and notified the parents of the other girls involved. He was concerned that these pictures could jeopardize college admission or future employment. He wanted his daughter to have more self-respect.

a. What do you think about the girls taking these types of pictures and circulating them among friends?

b. What do think about how the father reacted?

c. In your opinion, are these types of pictures embarrassing? Why or why not?

d. What are the limitations of privacy controls?

Example 2: While at a college party, a male/female couple went into one of the dorm rooms, assuming that the location afforded privacy. When he asked "Did you lock the door?" she answered "Yes." They began making out, fully clothed, oblivious to their surroundings. Unbeknownst to them, someone at the party had set up a camera in the room, which captured their private moment, and later posted the video via Vine, the social media service that shows 6-second video clips on a repeated loop. The next week at school, they were overwhelmed by the number of people who had seen the clip. Many were only too happy to show the offending video as they passed through the hallways. This couple was subjected to teasing and joking about an experience that was intended to be private.

a. What could this couple have done differently to insure privacy?

b. How do you feel about hiding cameras and circulating videos without consent?

c. How could someone have managed to record their private moment?

d. How might the boy have reacted to this situation? The girl's reaction? How would *you* have felt?

e. Would it make a difference if the couple involved were either lesbian or gay? Explain.

Example 3: Three boys decided to take a group photo, displaying themselves nude. They planned to send the photo to their girlfriends who were away at a softball tournament. They used the Snapchat app, set to delete the photo 10 seconds after its receipt, to prevent widespread circulation. One of the girls reacted quickly, asking a nearby friend to photograph her phone, thus saving the nude image which was clearly visible on her phone screen. The girls then had a copy of the image that eventually went viral. A photo that was intended to be private became very public.

a. What do you think about the boys sending a nude picture of themselves?

b. What do you think of the girls circulating the picture?

c. What are the pros and cons of using Snapchat?

d. In your opinion, how embarrassing do you believe this incident was for the boys involved?

e. What could the boys have done differently?

Tips for Staying Safe Online*

1. If you have an account on Facebook, regularly check the privacy controls because the options are periodically updated. Make sure your profile is shown only to your "friends" — not their friends too. You do not want your personal information to be circulating freely from person to person.

2. Do not be tempted to accept a friend request from a person you do not know.

3. Do not transmit anything on the Internet without knowing that anyone, anywhere could potentially see it. Once you transmit something, it then becomes irretrievable, and there is no guarantee that the person you sent it to won't forward it to others. **If it's private, don't post it!**

4. Never give out your name, address or phone number to unknown people, unless your parents have agreed that it is safe (e.g., for a delivery of an online order).

5. Make sure you have installed a password on your phone, or any other device that you use. Lock down your devices when you are not using them. Do not give out your password to your friends.

6. Do not click on suspicious-looking links. If something looks suspicious (e.g., it is from an unfamiliar website), delete it, or check with a teacher or parent before opening it.

7. If you think a message is from a friend but it looks strange or unlike something your friend might send, ask your friend about it before opening it. It is possible that someone else is using your friend's account to start trouble.

8. Always log out! Make sure you do not leave any account open when you go away from your phone, computer or other device. Friends who ask to borrow your phone or computer have access to your personal information. If you lend a device, do not give out your password — enter it yourself. Make sure you are OK with what the person plans to use your device for, and watch to see if they are being true to their word.

9. Make your password difficult to crack. Use a mixture of upper and lower case letters, and use both letters and numbers.

10. If something makes you uncomfortable or looks suspicious, tell a parent or teacher, or report it to the website you were trying to use.

---

* Adapted from Naked Security. (February 5, 2013). 10 tips to keep your kids and teens safe online. Retrieved August 22, 2014 from http://nakedsecurity.sophos.com/2013/02/05/top-10-tips-kids-safe-online

YOU CAN'T GET IT BACK

By Margo DeNuccio and Meghan Benson, MPH, CHES[*]

Objectives

By the end of this lesson, participants will be able to:

1. Describe three reasons why it is hard to "get something back" (both literally and figuratively) once they have texted or posted it online.

2. Identify at least three things to consider before texting or posting something online.

Rationale

In recent years, there have been many media stories about teens and young adults (and adults, too!) who have sent and posted pictures, videos and other content and later regretted doing so. Young people's stories often ended up as media headlines due to the extreme consequences of their behavior, including damaging friendships and dating relationships, losing jobs, being charged with crimes, and having to leave school due to widespread and constant bullying. Some of the saddest of these stories end with young people committing suicide because of something they or another person sent or posted about them.

While most young people do not experience such extreme consequences from sending or posting inappropriate content, many young people still engage in this behavior, which at the very least puts them at risk for later feeling uncomfortable or vulnerable or gets them in trouble at home or school. Young people may send or post content — such as rumors about others or nude pictures of themselves — then later regret doing so for some of the following reasons:

- They do not always consider the short- or long-term consequences of their actions.
- They do not think about how easily content can spread online and via cellphones.
- They get caught up in the emotions they are feeling at that moment (e.g., angry, upset, sexy, or excited).

Materials

- Flip chart or board, markers
- Index cards (at least one for each participant)

---

[*] Margo DeNuccio is the community outreach coordinator and Meghan Benson, MPH, CHES, is the director of community education for Planned Parenthood of Wisconsin, Inc.

- A packet for each student containing pieces of paper with images of various objects. Images can be taken from the **Educator Resource: Images for Participant Packets** or you can use your own images. Do not staple the papers; participants will be instructed to trade some images if they wish.

  Note:
  Not all packets have to contain the same number of images or the same images in them. Some may have just a couple images while others may contain many. Some may contain pieces of paper with all the same image while others may contain papers with all different images.

- "Sex and Tech: 5 Things to Think about Before Pressing Send," downloaded from http://thenationalcampaign.org/sites/default/files/resource-supporting-download/sex_and_tech_5_things.pdf

Procedure

1. Provide each participant in the group with a packet of images. Instruct participants not to open the packets until told to do so.

2. Tell participants that today the group will be discussing and completing activities dealing with the topics of texting, posting online and social media.

3. Have participants raise their hands if they have a phone and text at least once a week. Have participants raise their hands if they have a Facebook or other social media profile/account. If lots of participants raise their hands, be sure to acknowledge that this is a large percentage of the group.

4. Have participants raise their hands if they have ever sent a text or posted something and later regretted doing so or wished they could it take back. Be sure to indicate that they do not need to share what they specifically texted or posted.

5. Tell participants that while cell phones, texting and social media can be wonderful tools that make it easier to access information as well as communicate and connect with people, it is important to know how to use them responsibly.

6. Instruct participants to open their packets and take a moment to look at the images contained in them.

7. Instruct participants to walk around the room and exchange or trade images with their fellow participants as they wish. You should allow participants five to seven minutes to do this. Some

participants may have a particular strategy in exchanging images; that's OK. *(Maybe some want all of the images in their packet to be different. Others may want to collect pieces of paper with the same image on them. Some may want to collect as many different images as possible. Some may want to give away as many images as possible or none at all.)*

8. After participants have had five to seven minutes, choose several of the participants and give them each a piece of paper with one of the images from the packets on it. Explain to them that their responsibility is to retrieve all pieces of paper with that image on them. To do this, each participant will have to ask each fellow participant individually for their papers with that particular image on it. Give participants about five minutes to complete this task.

9. Explain to participants that texting something or posting something online is a lot like trying to get pieces of paper with certain images on them back once you have given them away.

   Discussion Questions:

   a. What were your feelings as you were handing out, collecting or trading the different images? (*Possible responses may include: "It felt fun — I didn't really think much about it," "I was focused on collecting or giving away certain images," "I kept wondering what the next step would be because I didn't know what we were going to do end up doing with the images. I didn't know what it meant."*)

   b. When you gave away or traded an image, was there any way you could control whether or not that images was shown or traded to other people in the group by the person you gave it to? How is this like texting something or posting something online?

   c. Is there anyone who decided not to trade, give away or accept any images at all during the activity? Why did they make the decision not to trade or collect images?

   d. For those participants who were responsible for getting pieces of paper with certain images back, was it difficult? Why was it difficult? How is this like trying to take or get back something you have texted or posted online?

10. Have participants brainstorm things they think are important to think about or consider before texting or posting something online. Write participants' responses on the board/flipchart.

    Possible responses or ideas may include: *How what you say/write is going to make others feel; if you are going to get in any trouble (legal or otherwise) for things that you post; if you are posting something that you would be willing to say to someone's face; whether or not you are being pressured by someone else to post/text something; if what you are texting is graphic or explicit, you can't change your mind/get something back once you've sent/posted it, etc.*

11. Give each participant a copy of the handout "Sex and Tech: 5 Things to Think about Before Pressing Send." Instruct participants to read over the handout to themselves and allow them five to seven minutes to do this. Or, call on various participants to read out loud one of the "things to think about" from the handout until each of them have been read.

12. Lead participants in a discussion about on the "things to think about" from the handout.

    Discussion Questions:

    a. What are your first reactions to this list? Are there any "things to think about" that you feel are more important than others?

    b. Have any of you ever been in a situation or know someone who has been in a situation where they have sent or posted something and then regretted doing so? What problems did this cause? How do you think that situation would have turned out better had the person considered some of the things on this list?

    c. Are there any "things to think about" you would add to the list?

    d. Will these tips change the way that you communicate via text, email or posting online? If so, in what ways?

13. Provide each participant with an index card and ask everyone to write down one thing they have learned or have been pushed to think more about after participating in the activity and discussion. Collect the index cards.

Images for Participant Packets

Copy and cut these images so that a single image is on a quarter-sheet of paper. Use these images when preparing participant packets (or use your own images).

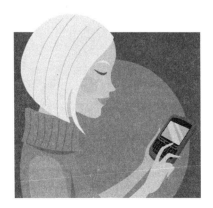
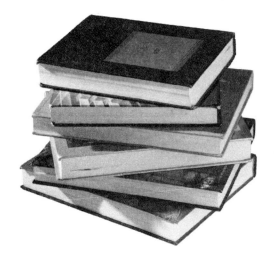

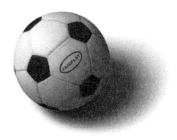
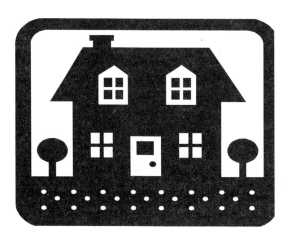

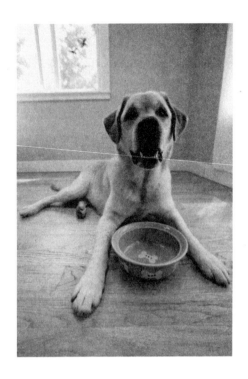

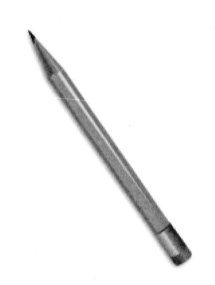

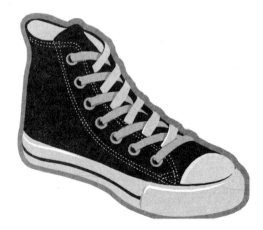

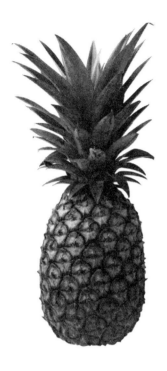

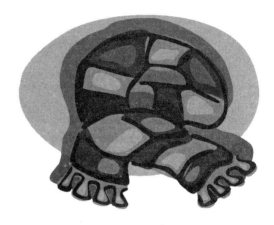

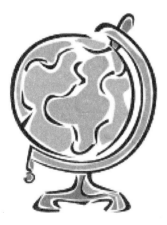

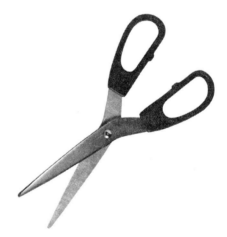

TEXT THEN SEXT ... WHAT HAPPENS NEXT?[1]

By Rebecca Roberts, MEd, CHES and Catherine Dukes, PhD[*]

Objectives

By the end of this lesson, participants will be able to:

1. Identify two common myths and facts about sexually explicit media.

2. Discuss two potential outcomes of sexting.

3. Apply a decision-making model to a sexting scenario.

Rationale

Recently, the topic of sexting and sexually explicit media (SEM) has become more common in sexuality education. As students become more wired to technology, exploration with sexuality within these media is more common, sometimes with unforeseen consequences. With an emphasis on sexting, cellphone use and the Internet, this lesson will allow participants to discover the myths and facts about SEM through an interactive game and case studies. Small-group processing will assist students in exploring these topics in greater depth, while enhancing decision-making skills and reflecting on personal beliefs and values.

Materials

- Flip chart paper, markers, tape
- **Educator Resource: Myths & Facts about Sexting**
- **Educator Resource: Looking at Some Sexting ... Scenarios**
- **Handout: Sexting Decisions**

Procedure

1. Title and post three sheets of flip chart paper as follows:

   MEDIA   **EXPLICIT**   **SEXUAL**

---

[1] Adapted with permission from Brick, P., Charleton, C., Kunins, H., & Brown, S. (2012). *Teaching Safer Sex, 3rd ed.* Taverner, B., Milstein, S., & Montfort, S. (Eds.). Morristown, NJ: The Center for Family Life Education.

[*] Rebecca Roberts, MEd, CHES, is the former education and training manager at Planned Parenthood of Delaware. Catherine Dukes, PhD, is the vice president of education and training at Planned Parenthood of Delaware.

Fold over the flip chart sheets so that the word on each sheet is covered. Then, unfold the first flip chart sheet and ask participants to give examples of **MEDIA.** Record participants' answers on the flip chart sheet.

2. Continue with the next flip chart sheet and ask participants what **EXPLICIT** means. Record their responses on the flip chart sheet. If participants have difficulty defining *explicit,* suggest that it means "clearly expressed" or "leaving nothing implied," such as "explicit instructions."

3. Finally, uncover the last flip chart sheet and ask participants what **SEXUAL** means. Record their responses.

4. After participants have come up with several descriptive words and examples for each flip chart sheet, praise them for their creativity. Next, change the title of **SEXUAL** to **SEXUALLY** and re-arrange the three sheets so that they read **"SEXUALLY EXPLICIT MEDIA."**

5. Ask for a few volunteers to define the term. Then read this definition:

   Sexually explicit media depicts uncensored sexual content. Examples include but are not limited to photography, illustrations, video and writing. The term *sexually explicit media* (SEM) is often used interchangeably with terms like *pornography* and *erotica.* SEM may include nudity, sexual intercourse and other sexual acts. SEM is difficult to define because what is or is not considered "sexually explicit" varies from person to person and culture to culture.

   Explain that for the rest of the lesson, you will be using the acronym "SEM" to refer to sexually explicit media.

6. Introduce a "word web" by writing **SEM** in the middle of the board or on a flip chart sheet. Draw a circle around it, with lines coming out of the circle, like a sun. Ask participants to think of **examples** of SEM, and **places** where a person might find SEM (e.g., magazines, fine art, educational or medical material, the Internet, museums). Record their responses on the lines all around the circle. Make sure to add **SEXTING** (sending sexually explicit images or messages over text) to the word web.

   Discussion Questions:

   a. Why does SEM exist?

   b. What are your thoughts or feelings about SEM?

    c. Now we're going to discuss sexting specifically. Why do some people sext?

    d. What are your thoughts or feelings about sexting?

    e. How do you think adults in your life feel about sexting? Why do you think they feel that way?

8. Tell participants that they will now have an opportunity to play a game in which they will examine myths and facts about SEM and sexting. Divide the class into two teams and have each team choose a team captain. Explain that you will take turns reading statements to each team and when it is their team's turn, they are to decide if the statement is a **MYTH** or a **FACT.** The team captains will be the only ones allowed to respond on behalf of their teams, and they will need to give a reason why the statement is a **MYTH** or **FACT.** Points will be awarded as follows:

- 1 point if the team responds correctly.
- 1 additional point if the team correctly explains why the statement is a **MYTH** or **FACT.**

9. Read the first statement from the **Educator Resource: Myths & Facts about Sexting** to the first team and give the team a few moments to discuss before asking the team captain for a response.

10. Continue by posing the next question to the second team, and continue alternating until all questions have been read. Declare the winning team and praise participants for their insight and ideas.

    Discussion Questions:

    a. Did any of the myths or facts surprise you? Explain.

    b. Why do you think myths about SEM persist?

11. Tell participants they will now have an opportunity to read and assess case studies in which teens encounter SEM. In their small groups they will discuss and decide the answers to a series of questions around the teens' thoughts, feelings, actions and possible consequences.

12. Divide participants into groups of about four to five participants and give each group one of the case studies from the **Educator Resource: Looking at Some Sexting ... Scenarios** and the **Handout: Sexting Decisions.** Participants will read the case study together and then answer the questions on the handout. When finished, groups will read their scenario to the large group and report their answers.

Discussion Questions:

a. Did these case studies seem realistic or unrealistic? Explain.

b. What were some of the feelings the characters had as they watched or sent SEM?

c. When your groups imagined what would happen next, were these mostly positive or mostly negative possibilities? Explain.

d. What might be some consequences of accessing sexually explicit media?

Note:

Possible consequences in the stories presented include: Criminal charges for possession of sexual images of a minor; widespread distribution of personal images without one's knowledge; feelings of embarrassment, shame or poor body image; being "in trouble" with one's parents; computer viruses, etc. Acknowledge also that a person might be fortunate and experience no negative consequences.

e. Do you think these consequences could happen to teens your age? Why or why not?

f. Why do you think some teens access SEM even if they are aware of the consequences?

g. How might a person avoid experiencing negative consequences of accessing SEM?

h. Which of the advice you heard would you recommend to your own friends?

13. Thank participants for their participation and thoughtful responses.

Myths & Facts about Sexting

1. **"Sexting" is harmless flirting.**

   MYTH. The material received may not be wanted by the other person. In addition, there are serious legal consequences when sexting involves minors under 18.

2. **Once you create a digital image of yourself and send it or post it online, you can no longer guarantee control of that image.**

   FACT. Unfortunately, you have no control over where your images or messages wind up. Images can be reproduced, forwarded, uploaded, etc. without a person's knowledge.

3. **Minors caught "sexting" can be charged with possessing or distributing child pornography.**

   FACT. There have been reported cases where young people sexting nude images have been charged with possession of child pornography, sometimes resulting in teens being required to register as sex offenders.

4. **All pornography is covered by First Amendment (free speech) rights.**

   MYTH. The Supreme Court has ruled some pornographic content is against the law, and that states have the right to restrict access to sexual content by minors.

5. **Taking a nude picture of yourself and sending it to your boyfriend or girlfriend is within your personal rights.**

   MYTH. It is against the law to send or be in possession of nude images of a minor (someone under the age of 18).

6. **Most television shows for general audiences contain references to sex.**

   FACT. Research has found that 70% of television programs for general audiences contain references to sex.

7. **Most people won't see any sexually explicit media until they become legal adults.**

   MYTH. Actually, research indicates that 70% of teens have come across pornography online accidentally.

8. **Taking or sending nude pictures of teens who are under the age of 18 can be considered creating and/or distributing child pornography *even if you are taking pictures of yourself.***

    FACT. Whether or not the pictures are of yourself or someone else, if you are in possession of nude images of someone under the age of 18, you may be at risk of legal consequences related to child pornography laws.

9. **Bare breasts are considered sexually explicit.**

    MYTH or FACT. Though different cultures define what "sexually explicit" means in different ways (MYTH) in the United States, bare breasts, buttocks and genitals are generally considered sexually explicit (FACT).

    Note:
    Whether the student says MYTH or FACT, have them explain their answer. The answer to this statement could be MYTH or FACT depending on the rationale given by the student.

10. **Receiving a nude or partially nude picture of a minor and forwarding it to others can have the same consequences as creating and sending your own sexually explicit photo.**

    FACT. Being in possession of a nude picture of a minor, whether you created it or received it, can have legal, social/emotional and/or school-based consequences.

Sources:
Kaiser Family Foundation. (2005). *Sex on TV 4.* Menlo Park, CA: Kaiser Family Foundation.

Peters, I. (2003). *Pornography: Discussing sexually explicit images: An Interactive learning guide for sexuality and health educators.* Seattle, WA: Planned Parenthood of Western Washington.

Pew Internet & American Life Project. (2005). *Protecting teens online.* Washington, D.C.: Pew Internet & American Life Project.

Lenhart, A. (December 15, 2009). *Teens and sexting.* Retrieved July 22, 2014 from
http://www.pewInternet.org/Reports/2009/Teens-and-Sexting/Overview.aspx

Looking at Some Sexting ... Scenarios

Scenario 1: *Jamie,* 17, has been dating *Alex,* 15, for six months. They go to different high schools and frequently text throughout the day. One day Alex decides to send a partially nude photo to Jamie. Two months later, Alex and Jamie break up. Jamie is angry and is thinking about forwarding the photo of Alex to some friends.

Scenario 2: *Dez,* 14, is chatting online with friends when someone sends a picture of a naked body with the face covered. Everyone is making jokes and commenting on the picture, trying to guess who it is. Someone dares Dez to send it to Jaylin, another student in their Biology class. Dez doesn't really want to but feels pressured and sends it anyway.

Scenario 3: *Chris,* 18, and *Rowan,* 18, have been dating for two years and sometimes sext each other. One day Rowan shows a nude picture of Chris to a close friend, Renée. Rowan leaves the room for a moment and Renée forwards the picture to her email and then sends it to some of her friends. People now make rude comments whenever Chris walks by. Chris is not sure why.

Scenario 4: *Izzy,* 17 and *Sidney,* 16 are at a party one Saturday night. Some of the teens are drinking. Later in the evening Izzy notices some teens are taking pictures of each other partially naked. On Monday morning, Izzy and Sidney receive some pictures of the kids at the party. Izzy thinks the pictures are pretty funny and wants to send them to some other friends. Sidney is a little uncomfortable and is not sure about sending the pictures. Sidney is also not sure if the kids in the pictures know these pictures are being shared.

Sexting Decisions

Directions: Read the case study assigned to your group, and then answer the following questions.

1. Why do you think the people in this story chose to sext? How do you think they felt at the time?

   _____

   _____

2. What do you think will happen next?

   _____

   _____

3. If the teens could go back in time and do it all over again, would they have made the same decisions about sexting? Why or why not?

   _____

   _____

4. What might people want to think about before taking and/or sending nude/semi-nude pictures?

   _____

   _____

5. What advice would you give your friends about sexting?

   _____

   _____

   _____

   _____

THINK BEFORE YOU TEXT

By Carolyn Cooperman, MA, MSW

Objectives

By the end of this lesson, participants will be able to:

1. Describe the importance of applying thought and restraint to text messages containing sexual content.

2. Use specific criteria for evaluating the appropriateness of a text message.

Rationale

According to a national survey, median text-using teenagers send 60 texts per day.[1] For today's adolescents, text messaging is a lifeline to friends. The non-stop, back-and-forth exchange through cyberspace is this generation's form of dialogue. The impulse to text is generally automatic and spontaneous, without much thought given to the content of a communication. The goal of this lesson is to help teens become more discriminating about the messages they decide to transmit. Since most texts circulate without adult oversight, it becomes especially important that teens develop skills for monitoring their own communications.

As text messages involving sexual content are explored, the opportunity to apply criteria such as truthfulness, privacy and tolerance brings another level of meaning to this exercise. By noting the special consideration that sex-related texts require, the bar is raised for viewing sexuality in a more complex and well-defined manner.

Materials

- Flip chart paper or board, markers
- **Handout: Writing Text Messages**

Procedure

1. Explain that the first part of the lesson simulates what can happen to a text message that circulates widely. Write the following example of an exchange of text messages on the board/flip chart:

---

[1] Lenhart, A. (March 19, 2012). *Teens, smartphones & texting.* Retrieved July 23, 2014 from
http://www.pewInternet.org/Reports/2012/Teens-and-smartphones.aspx

Cathy: Cn I borrow money for BC pills?

Mary: y do u need BC pills?

Cathy: I might do it

Mary: with who?

Cathy: none of ur business

Discussion Questions:

a. What went wrong in this texting conversation?

b. How might Cathy feel now?

c. How might Mary feel?

d. What would you do next if you were Mary? Cathy?

2. Explain that everyone will now write their own sample text messages as a follow up to the exchange that transpired between Cathy and Mary. Divide the group into pairs and distribute the **Handout: Creating Text Messages.** Instruct them not to put their names on the handout.

Allow time for the participants to complete the assignment. Collect the handouts, shuffle them, and redistribute them among the different pairs. Ask the participants to read aloud the sample texts that were written on the handouts.

3. Process this initial exercise with a group discussion.

Discussion Questions:

a. What is your opinion about how Mary used text messaging?

b. In what way is Cathy responsible for the problems that ensued?

c. Can you find any examples of hurtful or judgmental comments among the texts that we generated? Which ones were supportive?

d. Did any of the sample texts show restraint about participating in gossip?

e. Could the texts made by members in our group be considered truthful?

    f.   Of the sample texts that circulated today, which did you find most offensive? Why? Which text was your favorite? Why?

4.   The next part of this exercise begins to draw distinctions between texts that are written spontaneously, and those that are measured against a specific set of standards.

Write the criteria listed below on the board/flip chart. The discussion questions will help to exemplify the meaning of the terms, and show how they can be used as a mechanism for creating texts that are self-protective and considerate of others.

Things to Think about Before Texting
- **Public or Private**
- **Helpful or Hurtful**
- **Tolerant or Judgmental**
- **Truth or Rumor**

Discussion Questions:

    a.   What kind of sexual information do you believe should be kept private? What are some of the potential consequences that occur when private information becomes public?

    b.   Do you feel obligated to protect the privacy of others? Why, or why not?

    c.   If you knew a text would be hurtful before you sent it, what might motivate you to send it anyway? What would keep you from sending it?

    d.   Is there anything you would change about the spontaneous texts we wrote earlier, after considering some of these guidelines?

5.   Reshuffle the handouts of the sample texts that were written earlier, and redistribute them once again among small groups of two to three people.

Working from the list of **Things to Think about Before Texting,** have the participants apply the criteria to the text messages that were previously generated. To complete the assignment, they should write **Like** or **Dislike** to indicate their opinions about how the criteria were applied, and be prepared explain their thinking.

6.   Reconvene and review their results.

Discussion Questions:

a. In real-life situations, what would make you stop to think before sending a sex-related text?

b. How did you feel about participating in this exercise?

c. Can you see yourself using the recommendation to think before you text? Why, or why not?

Writing Text Messages

Directions: You and your partner will write your own sample text messages that relate to the exchange that transpired between Cathy and Mary.

First, you should know that Cathy stopped replying to Mary's texts because she felt that they were getting too personal. Mary got annoyed and sent the text below to many people at school:

Cathy finally did it!

Imagine that you and your partner for this exercise received Mary's text, and now will text each other about it. Use the space below to alternate making entries, as if you were actually texting. Start your conversation with:

Do u think she really did?

SAFER CYBER SEX
Exploring Online Relationships[1]

By Jessica Shields, CHES[*]

Objectives

By the end of this lesson, participants will be able to:

1. Describe the benefits and possible safety concerns of using the Internet.

2. Identify ways to use the Internet responsibly.

3. Explain how the Internet might enhance relationships and sexual experiences.

Rationale

The Internet is an ever-growing source of sexuality information and misinformation. People use the Internet to form relationships, get medical advice or information, create sexually expressive diaries, explore erotica, or to educate themselves. Many hours are spent surfing the Web, sending and receiving email, utilizing social networks, chat rooms and blogs, being a part of online discussions, or shopping and browsing websites. With the Internet as a dominant resource, it is important to take precautions against intrusions and fraud, including those that involve relationships. The purpose of this lesson is to help young adults feel more comfortable using the Internet responsibly to form relationships and access sexuality information.

Materials
- Flip chart paper or board, markers, pencils and tape
- **Handout: 10 Tips for Savvy Internet Use**
- **Handout: Cyber Situations**
- **Handout: Getting Personal**

---

[1] Adapted and reprinted with permission from Brick, P., Lunquist, J., Sandak, A., & Taverner, B. (2009). *Older, wiser, sexually smarter.* Morristown, NJ: The Center for Family Life Education.

[*] Jessica Shields, CHES, is a sexual health educator and trainer at Planned Parenthood of Central and Greater Northern New Jersey.

Procedure

1. Explain that the Internet can be a useful source for relationships and sexuality information. However, along with the advantages of the Internet, there may also be some disadvantages. Write **BENEFITS** and **POSSIBLE PROBLEMS** on separate sheets of flip chart paper or board and ask participants to brainstorm the benefits and possible problems of using the Internet as a resource for sexual information. Write the responses on the appropriate sheets or board. The lists might appear as follows. Supplement ideas as needed to spur discussion.

BENEFITS	POSSIBLE PROBLEMS
You can ...	*But ...*
Meet new people	You might not really "know" the other person
Get answers to your questions	Information might be inaccurate
Learn new information	Someone could take advantage of you
Talk to a partner far away	Scams
Express yourself freely	Stalkers
Be anonymous	Is real intimacy possible online?
Try new and different things	Too many sites — hard to navigate
Portray a different persona	It's impersonal

Discussion Questions:

a. What stories have you heard regarding online relationships?

b. Do people tend to think about the benefits or possible problems when discussing sex and online relationships? When accessing health information and advice? Explain.

2. Note that there are some simple things people can do to avoid possible problems while searching for intimacy, advice or information online. Ask participants for some precautions people can take to avoid problems.

3. Distribute **Handout: 10 Tips for Savvy Internet Use** and pencils, and briefly review each tip. Ask participants to work in pairs, and to evaluate the tips by placing stars next to the three tips they think give the BEST advice.

Discussion Questions:

a. Which tips are most important? Why?

b. Which tips do you think people would be most likely to follow? Why?

c. Why might a person decide not follow some of these tips?

d. What could you do to encourage someone you care about to follow any of these tips?

4. Explain that the Internet allows people to socialize, build friendships and relationships, seek advice, get information and discuss sexual issues. However, there are people who join online discussions or websites in order to victimize, harass or bully. In this next activity participants will review scenarios involving online situations.

5. Distribute **Handout: Cyber Situations.** Divide participants into small groups of about four people and assign each group one case study. Allow approximately 10 minutes for groups to discuss their cases and complete the handout. Suggest that they use the **Handout: 10 Tips for Savvy Internet Use** as a guide for help, if needed.

6. After 10 minutes, ask a representative from each group to read their group's case study aloud and summarize the group's discussion.

    Discussion Questions:

    a. How easy or difficult was it to complete the handout?

    b. How realistic are the situations? Explain.

    c. How helpful were the tips in examining the scenarios?

    d. Would you do anything differently the next time you go online? Explain.

7. Explain that posting an online personal advertisement is an easy way a person can meet others and form a relationship. Online personal ads provide a comfortable atmosphere where people can portray themselves in a positive and desirable way, frankly state what they want, and screen for their "type." Write the following sample websites on flip chart paper or board and explain that these resources provide links whereby a person can post a personal ad.

    www.eHarmony.com
    www.Match.com

8. Ask participants, "How many could imagine yourself using the Internet to find a partner?" and ask for a show of hands. Explain that even if they wouldn't, you hope they will have fun with this next activity creating a personal ad. Distribute **Handout: Getting Personal** and read the sample ad aloud. Tell participants that they may write the personal ad for themselves *or* for someone they know.

9. Allow participants about 10 minutes to write the personal ads. Afterward, ask for a few volunteers to read their ads to the group.

Discussion Questions:

a. What was it like to write a personal ad?

b. How easy or difficult was it to describe yourself?

c. Would you visit one of the websites listed? Why or why not?

d. Would you consider posting an ad online? Why or why not?

10 Tips for Savvy Internet Use

1 **PROTECT YOUR IDENTITY.** It could be risky to include your age, sex, address, place of work or places you visit on electronic correspondence. Create screen names and email addresses that are unidentifiable. Ask yourself: Who is asking? What information do they want? Why are they asking? What website am I visiting? How will the information I give be used?

2 **BE ALERT FOR SUSPICIOUS EMAIL.** Email is sometimes used to trick people into visiting websites that collect personal information, and downloading harmful software. Protect yourself by watching for unfamiliar emails, filtering unwanted email and keeping personal and financial information out of email messages.

3 **POST CAREFULLY.** When you put a photo, video or diary online, it can be seen around the world for a long time. Think about the information you have online, and whom you want seeing it. Avoid posting anything that you might regret, including sensitive personal data.

4 **KEEP YOUR PASSWORD PRIVATE.** Keep your email addresses and your Web pages private so only friends have access to them. Many social networking services (e.g., Facebook, Instagram) offer extensive privacy options. Use these settings to prevent anyone you don't know from viewing your information.

5 **CHAT AND EMAIL CAUTIOUSLY.** While chatting and emailing can be wonderful ways to start or maintain healthy relationships, it's important to use caution. Save copies of your online dating conversations. Only communicate with people whose addresses you recognize. If someone you don't know requests you as a contact, decline and block that person until you know who they are. Never give out personal information at the beginning. When you are ready to share more information, stick to first names and don't provide your full address. Ask questions that might help you determine if this person is legitimate. When you are ready to speak, start with a phone call and block your number.

6 **BE CAREFUL ABOUT MEETING YOUR "FRIENDS" IN PERSON.** If you are ready to meet an online "friend" in person, do so in a public place, during the day, and bring someone with you. Make sure a friend or family member knows where you are going and never leave or go home with your new friend.

7 **KNOW WHAT'S OUT THERE ABOUT YOU.** Go to a search engine, such as www.google.com, type in your name and see what other people might find if they conduct a search for you. By being aware of the information people see about you, you will be able to act accordingly.

8 **EVALUATE WEBSITES.** It is often difficult to differentiate between advertisements, trustworthy websites, opinion, credible information and misleading information. Learn search skills to get effective and accurate information. Use reliable directories and reputable websites as primary sources. Learn how to find and evaluate credible websites to limit unreliable information.

9 **USE SOFTWARE TO PROTECT YOUR COMPUTER.** Antivirus software, firewalls, and anti-spy programs can protect your computer from being violated. These programs protect your files, computer, and information from being accessed, copied, or ruined. Update these programs regularly to ensure continued protection.

10 **STAY INFORMED.** Know what to do and where to look if something goes wrong or if you suspect something may be wrong. Stay up to date and take action immediately to limit any damage that is done. Some helpful websites for further information include:
    www.ftc.gov
    www.getnetwise.org
    www.isafe.org
    www.staysafeonline.org
    www.wiredsafety.org

Sources:
www.cybersmart.org
www.staysafeonline.org
www.wiredsafety.org

Cyber Situations

Directions: In each of the following scenarios, a person is using the Internet for seeking a relationship or for accessing sexuality information. Discuss the situation with your group, and respond to the questions that follow. Use **Handout: 10 Tips for Internet Safety** to guide your discussions.

1 **Mark** just started dating someone new. He wants the relationship to become more physically intimate, but he is worried that he won't be able to please his new partner. Mark doesn't want to bother his doctor, but his friend told him about a natural herb he can take to enhance his erection. Mark found the herb online and wants to buy it. The company asked him to email his credit card information and address so the order can be processed.

Which tips from the handout would be most helpful for *Mark?* _____

What other advice would you give? _____

_____

2 Six months after her last long-term relationship ended, **Maria** decided that she was ready to start dating again. She started keeping a blog to cope with the challenges of finding the right partner and hopes other women can learn from her experiences. In her blog, you can find a picture of Maria and the name of the town where she lives. In her many blog entries, she has written about her dating experiences, her feelings, and things she's been doing for fun.

Which tips from the handout would be most helpful for Maria? _____

What other advice would you give? _____

_____

3 **Deidre** met someone online in a cooking chat room. Deidre thinks they have a lot in common and wants to continue to talk to this person.

Which tips from the handout would be most helpful for Deidre? _____

What other advice would you give? _____

_____

4 *Jean* and Josh met on an online dating website. Josh described himself as sweet, trustworthy and an animal lover. In his accompanying photo, he looked hot and was hugging a dog. Josh said he needed money for airfare so they could finally meet. Jean wired him $500 and they picked a date when they would finally meet. The next time Jean tried to e-mail Josh, the message was returned as undeliverable.

Which tips from the handout would be most helpful for Jean? _____

What other advice would you give? _____

_____

5 *Susan* and *Marquis* met online on a dating website. The two started chatting and soon began talking on the phone. When they finally met in person, it was mid-day at a local mall. The two have been happily dating for several months now.

Which tips from the handout would be most helpful for this couple? _____

What other advice would you give? _____

_____

Getting Personal

Directions: Create a personal ad for yourself or for someone else! Use the space below to draft your ad. It could include:

- The type of relationship you want (e.g., friendship, romance, companionship)
- Qualities you would like in a person (e.g., outgoing, non-smoking, athletic)
- Qualities you like about yourself (e.g., quiet, political, funny)
- Activities you enjoy (e.g., likes movies, enjoys cooking, digs gardening, etc.)

Sample Personal Ad

> *WOMAN SEEKING MAN*
>
> I am a hair designer from Southern California who would like to meet someone for more than the usual hook-up. I enjoy dining out, dancing, and long walks. My ideal partner would be a non-smoker, single guy between twenty-five and thirty-five who lives on the west coast, is willing to try new things, has a great sense of humor and loves dogs. No pressure! Let's just relax...become friends & get to know each other. E-mail me. I would love to chat with you.

Your Ad Here!

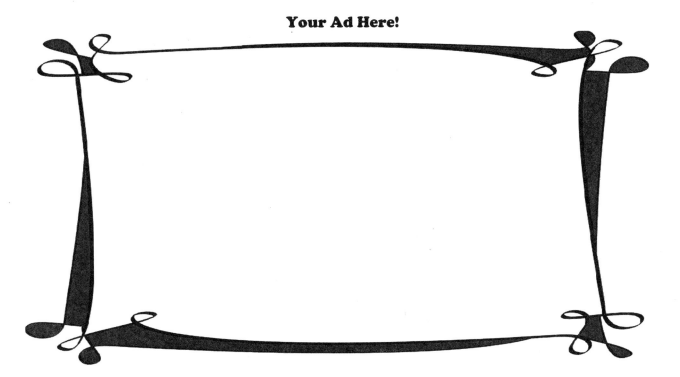

Now that you've gotten started, you might want to read other peoples' personal ads. Or you might even decide to post your own!

Section 6
Critical Decision Making in a Changing World

The heightened sexual sensations experienced by teens, particularly in the later adolescent years, often coincides with an increased interest in taking, transmitting and viewing pictures of a sexual nature. Since cameras are so readily available, and the taking of snapshots and videos is the way in which teenagers record everyday occurrences, it is not surprising that they often circulate sex-related pictures without giving much thought to the potential consequences involved.

The viewing of online pornography is another way that teens bring their hormone-driven needs into the technological arena. A manual on sex ed in the digital age would be remiss without offering both teachers and students guidelines for exploring the topic of pornography in a structured, academic manner, which have been reviewed by experienced sex educators from across the country. Whether or not schools, community groups and parents are ready to address the realities of our changing world by exploring this subject matter with mature high-school or college students will ultimately be decided by the communities involved. Lessons in this section include:

Porn, Porn Everywhere!:
A Values Clarification Lesson for Young Adults

Pornography, Online in the Digital Age

What Was I Thinking?

Decisions about Sexting

PORN, PORN, EVERYWHERE!
A Values Clarification Lesson for Young Adults

By Kirsten deFur, MPH[*]

Objectives

By the end of this lesson, participants will be able to:

1. Describe at least two opposing values about pornography that many people hold.

2. Identify at least three ways they will determine their personal values about pornography.

3. Articulate at least two factors that will help them make informed decisions about pornography.

Rationale

In this increasingly digital age, it is becoming easier and easier to access sexually explicit media such as pornography. Whether on a website, on a blog or on a smartphone, porn is just a click of a button away. Porn is, in essence, everywhere, which means that individuals will likely encounter it in some way, shape or form at some point in their lives. Few young people have had an opportunity to explore their values around something so ubiquitous. In addition, pornography is a hot-button issue, with a considerable amount of public and political discussion generating heated debates. Individuals need to be prepared to respond to pornography in healthy and productive ways, both when they encounter actual pornography and when they are confronted with the topic in society. One important part of preparing for that response is to examine personal values. This lesson will explore the many values that people hold regarding pornography, offer an opportunity for participants to evaluate their own values, and outline important factors to consider when making decisions about whether or not to consume pornography.

Materials

- Flip chart or board, makers, tape
- Blank paper and pens for the participants
- **Handout: I Think Porn Is ...** This handout has a Part 1 and Part 2, which should be copied on separate sheets of paper.

---

[*] Kirsten M. deFur, MPH, is a sexuality educator and trainer in Brooklyn, NY.

Procedure

1. Introduce the activity by stating that sexually explicit media appears in a wide variety of places. Ask participants to briefly share a few places that an individual might see sexually explicit media. *(Responses may include websites, blogs, magazines, movies, books, etc.)*

2. Point out that pornography exists in places that people may have to intentionally go to, and in places that people will stumble upon unintentionally. State that the goal of this lesson is to help the participants clarify their own values about pornography so that when they encounter sexually explicit media throughout their lives, they are able to make informed decisions about it. Read the following definition of the word *value* aloud, and instruct participants to keep it in mind as they discuss values: Values are "a person's principles or standards of behavior; one's judgment of what is important in life."[1]

3. Instruct the participants to turn to a neighbor to work together as pairs, and make sure each pair has a piece of paper and a pen. Tell the pairs to write down at least two opposing values related to pornography, and for each value, one source of where those values might originate from. After five to seven minutes, ask each group to share one of their values, and one of their responses regarding where that value comes from. Write the values shared on the board/flipchart. Allow each group to share.

   ### Discussion Questions:

   a. Where do our values about pornography come from?

   b. What is the range of values that people have about pornography? Is this beyond just pro and con?

4. Distribute Part 1 of the **Handout: I Think Porn Is ...** Instruct the participants to take 10 minutes to complete it independently, and let them know they will not be required to share their responses.

5. Once everyone is finished with Part 1, divide the group up into small groups of four or five participants. Distribute Part 2 of the handout to each small group and ask the participants to respond to the questions. Inform the groups that they will be asked to share highlights from their discussion. After 10 minutes, reconvene as a large group and review the questions on the Part 2 of the handout.

---

[1] Oxford University Press. (n.d.). Value. Retrieved July 23, 2014 from
http://oxforddictionaries.com/us/definition/american_english/value

Discussion Questions:

   a. What was your experience completing the handout like? What was challenging?

   b. How do people determine their values about porn?

   c. What is the importance of examining personal values about porn?

   d. How much do people's values impact whether or not someone accesses porn?

   e. How might you react to someone who articulated a value about porn that was very different from your own?

6. Ask the participants, "What factors are important when people make decisions about porn?" Write down responses on the board/newsprint. Responses may include personal values; style of porn (e.g., amateur, mainstream, feminist); if the performers have safe working conditions; if the sex that is portrayed is realistic; if a safer-sex method is used; if it will negatively impact one's relationship; if the subject has not consented to the image being shared publicly (e.g., "revenge porn"), etc.

Discussion Questions:

   a. What makes it difficult for people to determine their values about porn?

   b. What would make it easier for people to determine their values about porn?

7. Instruct the participants to get back into their small groups from the previous activity. Tell the groups to come up with a "Porn Checklist," which includes at least five things that an individual needs to decide before viewing pornography. Give the groups 5-10 minutes to complete their checklists. Ask each group to share one thing from their list.

Discussion Questions:

   a. How much do you think the average U.S. college student thinks about porn?

   b. How much do you think the average U.S. college student thinks about all these factors?

   c. How can the factors we discussed influence someone's porn consumption?

   d. How can you help your peers think more critically about porn?

I Think Porn Is ... (Part 1)

Directions: Complete this page independently, based on your own personal opinions. For each question, you must indicate whether you **Agree** or **Disagree** with the statement. You will not be required to share your responses.

	Agree	Disagree
1. Actors in pornographic films should be required to use barrier methods that protect against HIV and other sexually transmitted infections (STIs).		
2. If someone looks at pornography, it means they are not sexually aroused by their current partner.		
3. If someone watches pornography, it's best if they keep it private.		
4. Individuals who view too much porn will not have a healthy sexual relationship with another person.		
5. It's OK for an individual to want to perform in a pornographic scene.		
6. Once a couple decides to be monogamous, neither person should seek out sexually explicit material.		
7. People need to just accept that porn is a part of life, and not worry about who is watching whom do what.		
8. Pornography is degrading to women.		
9. The government should place more regulations on the porn industry.		
10. The sex shown in porn should always be clearly consensual and demonstrate the use of external or internal barrier methods such as condoms.		
11. There should be age restrictions placed on who can purchase sexually explicit material.		
12. Viewing pornography can be a healthy sexual experience when by yourself.		
13. Watching porn in secret will damage a relationship.		

I Think Porn Is... (Part 2)

Directions: As a small group, discuss your responses to the questions listed below. You will be asked to share highlights from your discussion with everyone.

1. How easy/difficult was it to complete Part 1? Why?

2. How did you decide if you agree or disagree with the statements?

3. What are some ways that you can determine what your values are regarding porn?

4. How much influence do our values have over our decision making?

PORNOGRAPHY, ONLINE IN THE DIGITAL AGE

By Carolyn Cooperman, MA, MSW

Objectives

By the end of this lesson, participants will be able to:

1. Make distinctions between the fantasies portrayed in pornography and the emotional and health-related realities confronted in actual relationships.

2. Understand the role that communication plays in sexual relationships.

3. Clarify misconceptions and misinformation about pornography.

Rationale

A Google search using the term *sex pictures* returns 83 million results in less than one-tenth of a second. With 93% of boys and 62% of girls reporting exposure to Internet pornography during adolescence, online viewing is considered to be a normative experience for the majority of teenagers.[1] Yet despite the increased availability and exposure to online pornography, corresponding opportunities for constructive discussions about this medium, with peers and informed adults, are unfortunately non-existent for most teens. When sexual topics are cut off from legitimate inquiry, negativity and secrecy is reinforced. The challenge for educators is to use strategies that turn the underground topic of pornography into a thought-provoking subject worthy of a serious investigation. This might include exploring gender differences regarding pornographic use, or the limitations of fantasy in real-life situations. Educators have the unique advantage of working with teens in peer settings where participants themselves take the lead in raising self-protective concerns.

Materials

- **Educator Resource: Commonly Asked Questions and Answers about Pornography**
- **Handout: Pornography: What It Includes and What It Leaves Out**
- **Educator Resource: Talking about Pornography.** Prior to the lesson, copy each of the four group assignments onto index cards. Make another identical set of cards if you are working with a large group.

---

[1] Sabina, C., Wolak, J., & Finkelhor, D. (2008). The nature and dynamics of Internet pornography exposure for youth. *CyberPsychology & Behavior, 11(6):* 691-693.

Procedure

1. Begin the lesson by asking the following questions: "How many of you have had the opportunity to talk about pornography in a classroom or group setting? Why do you think we are going to talk about it today?"

   Explain that discussions about pornography generally evoke strong reactions in people, ranging from very positive to very negative. Since some are familiar with online pornography and others are not, it is to be expected that opinions and practices related to this topic will vary considerably. Review ground rules that encourage respect for varying viewpoints.

   Note:

   For this topic, and others as well, some participants may prefer to raise their questions anonymously. A question box is a useful tool for eliciting their concerns. The **Educator Resource: Commonly Asked Questions and Answers about Pornography** offers suggestions for how to respond to the questions that are typically asked.

2. Divide the participants into small groups and distribute the **Handout: Pornography: What It Includes and What it Leaves Out.** Allow time for the participants to complete the assignment. Reconvene, review the responses, and follow up with a discussion.

   Discussion Questions:

   a. Which items on the list are primarily learned through **self-discovery?**

   b. Which items on the list can only be learned from **interaction with a sexual partner?**

   c. Since online pornography rarely models condom use, do you think viewers will become less vigilant about pregnancy and STI prevention? Explain.

   d. Which questions seemed to evoke agreement among members in your group? Disagreement? Explain why.

   e. Were there any gender differences in the ways in which males and females regard pornography? Explain.

3. This next exercise enables participants to have a more in-depth conversation about some of the issues that were introduced earlier in this lesson. Form new groups consisting of three to four participants and distribute one group assignment from **Educator Resource: Talking about Pornography** to each group. Allow time for the groups to complete the assignments that are listed on their cards, review their responses, and follow up with a group discussion.

Discussion Questions:

a. What important considerations about pornography and relationships were shared? Is there anything else to consider?

b. What advice would you give to a couple if one person wanted to view pornography online, and the other did not?

c. Did you find it helpful to talk about pornography? Why? Why not?

Commonly Asked Questions and Answers about Pornography

This material was developed for educator use and is not intended to be used as a handout for group participants. However, educators may want to raise some of these questions with their participants to better assess their knowledge and concerns.

Does pornography corrupt morals?

Lots of social constructs — religion and many cultural traditions — do object to pornography. And yet, pornography is ubiquitous. A 2013 report found that porn websites get more visitors than Amazon, Netflix and Twitter *combined.*[1] Pornography does not pretend to teach moral standards. Morality develops from the values instilled by parents, friends and the culture in which one lives. Most people watch pornography for self-stimulation, and this is common and not harmful. When a person has a high regard for self and others, and shows respect and consideration for the well-being of a sexual partner, these moral convictions can be maintained, regardless of whether a person watches pornography.

Should people watch pornography to learn how to have sex?

Pornography is a multi-billion dollar industry, the purpose of which is to make money. Adolescents primarily use pornography for self-stimulation, developing sexual awareness, and erotic purposes. **It is in no way intended to be used as a guide for teenage sexual relationships.**

Recent research shows that pornography may have some detrimental effects on young women, young men and same-sex attracted young people. Young women felt they needed to perform acts that pleased their partners; young men felt that they could not measure up to the male performers in pornography; and same-sex attracted young people objected to the dominant/submissive imagery that seemed to mirror heterosexual sex.[2] When any attempt to emulate pornographic imagery is forced, coerced or unpleasing, the action is experienced as unwanted and abusive.

Does pornography portray what sex is really like for most people?

In commercial pornography, sex acts are chosen for how they will look on camera. They do not generally portray what people want or need in real relationships. While the images may be erotic, pornographic sex is exaggerated and sensationalized. Pornography, outside of the context of a real relationship, leaves out the emotional aspects of sex that include affection and pleasure. Individuals

---

[1] The Huffington Post. (May 4, 2013). Porn sites get more visitors each month than Netflix, Amazon and Twitter combined. Retrieved July 23, 2014 from http://www.huffingtonpost.com/2013/05/03/internet-porn-stats_n_3187682.html

[2] Crabbe, M., & Corlett, D. (2010). Eroticizing inequality: Technology, pornography and young people. *DVRCV Quarterly, Edition 3, Spring 2010.* Retrieved July 23, 2014 from http://www.awe.asn.au/drupal/sites/default/files/Crabbe%20Corlett%20Eroticising%20Inequality.pdf

intuitively bring these emotional needs to their sexual relationships, which are triggered by the desire for closeness, affiliation and connection.

Does pornography lead to sexual violence?

Many people vehemently denounce pornography as being degrading to women and potentially responsible for inciting sexual violence. Many people refrain from viewing pornography for these reasons, and that is an understandable personal choice.

Current research, however, is demonstrating that in spite of the increased availability and exposure to the violent images found in online pornography, the incidence of rape and other sexual assaults has declined.[3] Additionally, teens are actually delaying the onset of their first sexual relationships and are more inclined to practice safer sex.[4]

Is watching too much pornography bad for you?

This is a complex question and deserves both validation for the normal adolescent curiosity and interest in pornography, as well as some of the potential risks involved with excessive viewing.

Teenagers have always been interested in viewing nudity and discovering their own sexual response through masturbation, and will seek outlets to relieve heightened sexual sensations. It is important to acknowledge these underlying needs as being normal and commonplace.

The primary concerns about early, prolonged pornographic use involve the possibility of using pornography compulsively to alleviate stress. Viewing pornography is not in itself harmful when the user can set limits. If compulsive viewing increases isolation or causes distress, help is available by discussing this problem with parents or a counselor. Additionally, pornography can reinforce negative attitudes about towards sex, women and unrealistic expectations about sex.

Are you more desirable sexually if you look like a porn star?

Porn stars are paid actors whose bodies have been altered to entertain. Exaggerated penis and breast size, the removal of pubic hair, or body types that are too good to be true are emphasized in pornography. Millions and millions of people all over the world who do not have "perfect" bodies find partners and engage in pleasurable, satisfying sex without altering their bodies. It would be a mistake to assess the normalcy of one's own body by using porn stars as role models.

---

[3] Chapman, S. (November 5, 2007). Is pornography a catalyst of sexual violence? Retrieved July 23, 2014 from http://reason.com/archives/2007/11/05/is-pornography-a-catalyst-of-s

[4] Castleman, M. (April 27, 2009). Does pornography cause social harm? Retrieved July 23, 2014 from http://www.psychologytoday.com/blog/all-about-sex/200904/does-pornography-cause-social-harm

Pornography: What It Includes and What It Leaves Out

Directions: For each of the items listed below, check **Yes** if it can be learned from pornography, **No** if it cannot be learned from pornography, and **Maybe** for mixed reactions to the item.

	Yes	No	Maybe
1. Possible ways of achieving sexual pleasure.			
2. How to talk about sex with a partner.			
3. Various types of sexual behavior.			
4. Common ways that most adults have sex.			
5. Types of images that might be shocking.			
6. How to say "no" to unwanted sexual behavior.			
7. Standards for how to treat a partner in a relationship.			
8. Images that might enable arousal and orgasm.			
9. How normal bodies generally look.			
10. Common ways that people have sex.			
11. What a partner will be willing to try.			
12. Safer-sex practices for preventing pregnancy and sexually transmitted infections (STIs).			
13. Sex involving an emotional connection to another person.			
14. What a real-life partner would find pleasing.			
15. The emotional effects of sexual violence.			
16. Signs that the men portrayed in pornography are sexually aroused.			
17. How to be a good sexual partner.			
18. A method for distinguishing fantasy from reality.			
19. A guide for how you would like sex to be in real life.			
20. Signs that the women portrayed in pornography are sexually aroused.			

Talking About Pornography

The exercise outlined below is meant to be experienced in small groups. Copy the group assignments listed below, then cut and paste each onto separate index cards. If you have a large group, make several sets of the same cards, allowing more than one group to complete the same assignment. This works well for comparing people's perceptions. However, each group should have only one card.

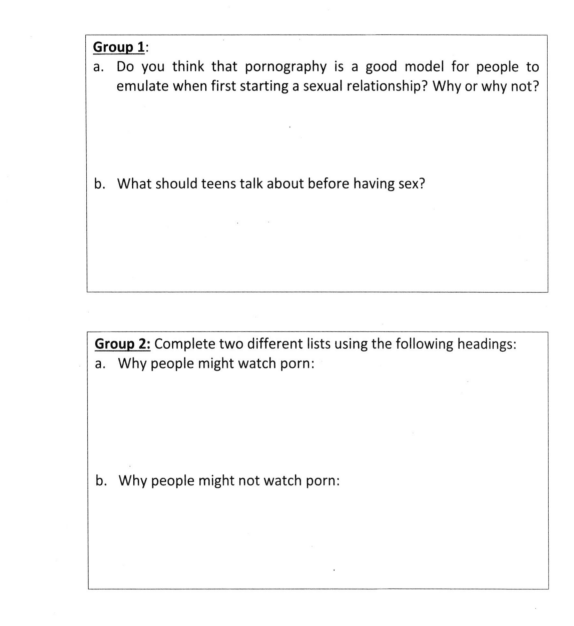

Group 1:
a. Do you think that pornography is a good model for people to emulate when first starting a sexual relationship? Why or why not?

b. What should teens talk about before having sex?

Group 2: Complete two different lists using the following headings:
a. Why people might watch porn:

b. Why people might not watch porn:

Group 3: Some might try to emulate pornographic sex in real relationships, but their partners might be unwilling. Pornography does not model how to say "no" to unwanted sexual behavior. List at least five different statements for saying "no" to sexual behavior that attempts to emulate pornography, but is unwanted by a partner. Put a check next to the statement that you think would achieve the most effective result.

Group 4: Pornography usually does not model the qualities that a good sexual partner should have.

a. List some of the qualities that you think a good sexual partner should have. (The group doesn't have to agree. It is OK to list varying viewpoints.)

b. What qualities in a sexual partner would be a turn-off? You can agree to disagree.

WHAT WAS I THINKING?

By Carolyn Cooperman, MA, MSW

Objectives

By the end of this lesson, participants will be able to:

1. Describe how different aspects of brain functioning can affect decision-making about sexting.

2. Explain that pleasure is regulated by brain chemistry and serves an important function for human survival.

3. Participate in a role-play that demonstrates how pleasure-seeking behavior and rational thought can come into conflict.

4. Apply knowledge about the relationship between the prefrontal cortex and dopamine chemicals to scenarios about sexting.

Rationale

On a cognitive level, adolescents are well aware that sexting or transmitting sexually explicit photos carries risk. Embarrassment, ridicule and admonishment from adults (e.g., parents, school officials, even police authorities) are all examples of potential consequences. Why then might teenagers leave themselves wide open to humiliation and public scrutiny?

There are times when approval from peers can outweigh the risks of engaging in a dangerous practice. Additionally, pleasure-seeking behavior, such as the excitement that occurs when picture taking becomes associated with sexual arousal explains why teens sometimes throw caution to the wind.[1] This lesson uses some very basic principles in neuroscience and applies them to decision-making about sexting. As the participants explore real-life dilemmas related to sexting, they gain a clearer understanding of the dynamics involved.

Materials

- Flip chart paper or board, markers
- **Handout: What Was I Thinking?**

---

[1] Schaffhausen, J. (November 26, 2000). The pleasure principle: Connections between reward and learning. Retrieved July 24, 2014 from http://brainconnection.brainhq.com/2000/11/26/the-pleasure-principle-connections-between-reward-and-learning

Procedure

1. Begin the lesson with two examples of pleasure-seeking experiences. Ask the participants: "Why do you think some people skydive even though they are well aware of the risks involved?" Tell them that skydiving, although dangerous, can elicit extreme feelings of pleasure, joy, success or euphoria. In spite of the risks, those who pursue skydiving do so because of the good feelings it evokes.

2. Next, have the participants create a mental image of a favorite food. Ask them to close their eyes to think more specifically about the image, paying attention to the smell, texture and appearance of that particular food.

   Discussion Questions:

   a. What sensations did the image of a favorite food evoke?

   b. Was the food you thought about known to be healthful or unhealthful?

   c. If it was an unhealthful food, would you still crave it, even in spite of what you know about its health-related properties?

   d. What is the biological advantage of making thoughts about food pleasurable? *(The pleasure associated with food motivates people to eat, which is necessary for survival.)*

   e. What is a disadvantage? *Overeating can lead to obesity.*

3. Conclude this exercise by stating that pleasure is a strong motivating force that is important for human survival. At times however, pleasure can motivate behavior that runs counter to self-interest, e.g., we eat too much.

   State that sex is another important biological function that is also associated with pleasure. Ask the participants: "What is the biological advantage of making sex pleasurable?" *Sex is pleasurable so that people will be motivated to reproduce.*

4. Explain that you will now focus on how sexting exemplifies the relationship between pleasure-seeking behavior and rational thought. Write the headings listed below on the board/flip chart:

   PREFRONTAL CORTEX   **DOPAMINE CHEMICALS**

5. Explain that the prefrontal cortex, or frontal lobe, is the **thinking part of the brain,** the part of the brain located behind the forehead. When people make decisions about whether or not to participate in sexting, this is the part of the brain that is used.

Ask the participants to make a list of the kinds of things that the rational part of the brain would be emphasizing about the potential consequences of sexting. List the contributions under the **PREFRONTAL CORTEX** heading.

Possible list: *Embarrassment, ridicule, parental disapproval, possible legal charges about transmitting or possessing nude pictures of minors (see note at end of lesson), goes against social norms that require nudity to be private, relationship problems (e.g., violation of trust should someone expose the pictures without consent), etc.*

6. Explain that dopamine chemicals are also referred to as **"feel-good chemicals."** These chemicals are produced in the brain and trigger the pleasurable sensations associated with food, drugs, cigarettes, sex, etc. Dopamine chemicals have nothing to do with rational thought. The feel-good chemicals are only concerned with motivating an individual to continue to pursue pleasure.

    Create a list of how dopamine chemicals would urge an individual to pursue sexting because sexting is associated with sexual arousal and feels good. List their contributions under the **DOPAMINE CHEMICALS** heading.

    Possible list: *This feels good, go for it, I need that picture, the picture will bring back the pleasurable feelings of sex, all I care about is the picture, I want that picture!*

7. Divide everyone into two groups. Provide the following instructions for enacting a group role-play:

    We are going to enact a group role-play that demonstrates how the **prefrontal cortex** and **dopamine chemicals** are at odds with one another when deciding about sexting. Half of you will play the role of the **"Prefrontal Cortex,"** and the other half will be **"Dopamine Chemicals."**

    Assign the roles and continue with the instructions:

    In the role-play, the prefrontal cortex will promote the **rational concerns** about sexting, and the dopamine chemicals will promote the **pleasurable motivations** for sexting. Refer to the lists that we just created to help you understand your role.

8. Allow a few minutes for the role-play. Follow up with a discussion.

    Discussion Questions:

    a. What was it like being the prefrontal cortex?

    b. What was it like being dopamine chemicals?

    c. Do you agree with any of the arguments that the prefrontal cortex promoted? Why, or why not?

    d. How do you feel about the arguments promoted by the dopamine chemicals?

    e. Would it be wise to make decisions about sexting while sexually aroused? Why, or why not?

9. Divide everyone into smaller groups and distribute the **Handout: What Was I Thinking?** This handout is designed to reinforce and expand upon the concepts that were previously introduced. Allow time for the groups to complete the handouts, review their responses to the assignment, and follow up with a discussion.

    Discussion Questions:

    a. Why do people sometimes take risks that leave them open to embarrassment or public humiliation?

    b. How are the examples on the handout similar? Different?

    c. What advice would you give to someone who was thinking about taking sexually explicit photos?

    d. What advice would you give to someone who was thinking about *sharing* sexually explicit photos?

    e. How might a person experience sexual pleasure without taking a picture? (*Refer back to the example of a food craving that was elicited without a photo.*)

Note:
Sending or possessing sexually explicit pictures of minors may violate child pornography laws in some states. Where this is the case, sexting between teens may be considered a felony. While many believe that minors should be distinguished from adults and should be charged more appropriately, check your state laws to find out about the statutes in your area. See http://www.sexetc.org/action-center/sex-in-the-states or check www.ncsl.org and search for "sexting legislation."

What Was I Thinking?

Directions: Read the examples below and answer the questions that follow.

Example 1: Lou has been asking his girlfriend Sabrina to send him a nude photo, and she has refused. His friends were quick to point out his lack of success, and insisted that if she were really into him, she would do this for him. They suggested that he compliment her for her looks, convince her of his own concerns for her reputation, and threaten to break up if nothing else worked. They took bets, and ultimately all bet against the likelihood that Lou would finally convince her. Weeks later Lou and Sabrina continued to be involved sexually, and one time, Sabrina went home and surprised Lou by sending a nude pic. In his excitement about getting the photo, he forwarded it to one of his friends as proof of his success. The pic eventually circulated around their school. Both Lou and Sabrina must have wondered, **"What was I thinking?"**

a.   What evidence can you find, if any, of **prefrontal cortex** functioning in this example?

b.   Were **dopamine chemicals** an influence? Explain why or why not.

c.   Is peer pressure a common influence on decision-making about sexting? Why or why not?

d.   Should this couple stay together? Why or why not?

Example 2: Olivia and Bess were in the habit of sending nude pics to one another via Instagram. They did this primarily to bring back memories of their sexual experiences, and usually deleted the photos immediately upon receiving them. They trusted one another, and had full confidence that neither one of them would expose these photos. The nature of their relationship was unknown in their school, however, they were growing increasingly tired of the secrecy. One night, they decided to send and keep a pic of themselves, fully clothed, but kissing. Unbeknownst to them, Olivia's brother borrowed her cell phone, found the pic, and forwarded it to a friend. The photo, as well as the news about their relationship, circulated the next day. Each must have asked herself, **"What was I thinking?"**

    a. How was the **prefrontal cortex** operating in this example?

    b. Were the **dopamine chemicals** at work? Explain.

    c. Could risk-taking about sexting be influenced by the prejudice and secrecy surrounding a person's sexual orientation? Explain.

    d. What advice would you give to the brother who exposed the photo?

    e. Should teens use telephone passwords? Why, or why not?

DECISIONS ABOUT SEXTING

By Carolyn Cooperman, MA, MSW

Objectives

By the end of this lesson, participants will be able to:

1. Identify and clarify personal beliefs about sexting.

2. Practice negotiation skills about sexting.

Rationale

According to recent research, one in ten children aged 10-17 has used a cellphone to send or receive sexually suggestive pictures.[1] The images they transmit tend to be less graphic than those that circulate among 18- to 19-year-olds. Nonetheless, news of sexting travels fast in school settings. Students react with interest, curiosity, shock and excitement. The exercises about sexting that are used in this lesson are meant to be fun and engaging, but they also challenge participants to identify personal beliefs, share thoughts with peers, raise uncertainties and clarify facts. Participants are asked to observe discrepancies in their own thinking (e.g., sexting may be seen as being both "fun" and "trouble"). Skills for defending beliefs and negotiating conflicts are practiced by working in small groups and participating in a role-play.

Materials

- **Handout: Thoughts about Sexting**

Procedure

1. Warm up with some questions about sexting: "Who can define sexting?" "How common do you think sexting is in this school?"

   Definition: For the purposes of this lesson, sexting, as practiced by teenagers, primarily consists of sending nude photographs or videos between mobile phones or other electronic media.

2. Distribute the **Handout: Thoughts about Sexting** and ask participants to complete it individually. When finished, divide the group into pairs to compare their results. State that not

---

[1] Mitchell, K.J., Finklehor, D., Jones, L., & Wolak J. (2012). Prevalence and characteristics of youth sexting: A national study. *Pediatrics, 129(1):* 13-20.

everyone will have the same beliefs, and encourage participants to explain the thoughts behind their responses. Some participants may want to change their responses after talking to others.

3. Ask the pairs to circulate once or twice more to compare responses with different sets of participants. Encourage them to talk to both males and females as they form different pairs so that they can assess possible gender differences in their responses. Reconvene and follow up with a discussion.

   ### Discussion Questions:

   a. Which statements seemed to generate agreement? Disagreement?

   b. Which statements raised uncertainty?

   c. What did you learn about sexting from talking to others? Did you learn anything that convinced you to change your mind?

   d. Did the males and females differ in their opinions about sexting?

   e. What should a person do when sexting is thought to be both "fun" and "trouble"?

   Note:
   Sending or possessing sexually explicit pictures of minors may violate child pornography laws in some states. Where this is the case, sexting between teens may be considered a felony. While many believe that minors should be distinguished from adults and should be charged more appropriately, check your state laws to find out about the statutes in your area. See http://www.sexetc.org/action-center/sex-in-the-states or check www.ncsl.org and search for "sexting legislation."

4. Tell participants they will be enacting a role-play to further explore some of the concepts introduced in the previous exercise. Explain that decisions about sexting may involve negotiation when there is uncertainty about whether to participate in sexting or differences exist between the parties involved. Read the role-play to the group:

   A 16-year-old couple, Dakota and Casey, have been dating for over a year. Dakota has asked Casey for a nude picture sent via Instagram. They like each other very much, but Casey wonders what to say to Dakota about this. Enact a possible conversation that might occur between them.

   Work with the group to explore possible things to negotiate (e.g., risks, doubts, reasons behind opinions, feelings about disagreement, showing respect for differences but sticking to a decision, etc.).

   As the role-play continues, ask for volunteers to step in and substitute for Casey and Dakota.

Note:

Participants might ask whether the characters are male or female. The names *Dakota* and *Casey* are intentionally androgynous, so that participants may focus on the quality of the conversation, not the characters' genders or sexual orientations. As such, substitutes may be of any gender or sexual orientation.

Repeat the role-play, but this time, change it so that Casey and Dakota are a gay or lesbian couple.

5. Follow up with a group discussion.

    Discussion Questions:

    a. What kinds of things did the couple discuss?

    b. Why were these things discussed?

    c. Do you think the conversation(s) went well? Explain.

    d. Do you think it mattered whether the couple was gay, lesbian or heterosexual? Why or why not?

    e. Can you see this happening in real life?

    f. Do you think the relationship can continue?

Thoughts about Sexting

Directions: For each item, check the box that best describes your opinion.

	Agree	Disagree	Unsure
1. Sexting is OK for people in love.			
2. It's fine to receive a nude photo, not to send one.			
3. I am not ready to make any decisions about sexting.			
4. Sexting is trouble.			
5. Sexting is OK for college students.			
6. It's not too difficult to take back a nude picture from the Internet.			
7. Break up with anyone who pressures you into sexting.			
8. Sexting is fun.			
9. The sending or possessing of nude pictures of minors should be illegal.			
10. Adults should be more open-minded about sexting.			
11. Taking a nude picture of a person without their consent is morally wrong.			
12. Sexting is risky.			
13. The majority of my friends would not send nude pictures of themselves.			
14. If I received a nude picture of one of my friends, I would delete it immediately.			

Section 7
Preparing Sex Educators and Parents for the Digital Age

Linking sex education and technology is an uncharted course for both educators and parents. In this new age, it is necessary to keep pace with the ways in which technological advancements are impacting teenage sexual development. The lessons offered in this section allow teachers and parents to think about, explore and experience electronic potential. The lessons provide a conceptual framework for how technological use and sexual learning are integrated.

When teachers and parents work cooperatively, we double the possibility of fostering sexual health in new and innovative ways. This important partnership is a cornerstone of effective sex education programs. Lessons in this section include:

Technology and Teenage Sexuality:
A Lesson for Parents

Helping Teens Act Purposefully in a Digital World:
A Lesson for Parents and Professionals

A 21st-Century Conversation Guide to
Teenage Sexuality and Technology:
A Lesson for Adults

TECHNOLOGY AND TEENAGE SEXUALITY
A Lesson for Parents

By Carolyn Cooperman, MA, MSW

Objectives

By the end of this lesson participants will be able to:

1. Understand the interplay between developing sexuality and technology use.

2. Make distinctions between harmful and beneficial technological practices.

3. Conduct online searches that can be of support to parents in the digital age.

Rationale

Teenagers basically launch themselves into the digital age. They are curious, creative, adventurous and sometimes daring as they experiment with the new technologies. The fascination with electronics occurs against the backdrop of accelerated sexual development. It therefore becomes logical and predictable that teens will bring their sex-related concerns into the technological arena. For their parents, adjusting to sexual development alone is sufficiently challenging. Now they must contend with the knowledge that what their children can search for online, who they contact, and what they transmit goes far beyond the boundaries that existed in the past.

Parents are a motivated group — there is a lot at stake. This lesson tries to strike a balance between addressing the legitimate safety concerns that parents have about the new technologies, while offering them an introduction into the types of technological resources that can actually benefit teenagers. Integrated throughout are opportunities for parents to consult with one another as they strive to define technological parameters in a rapidly changing world.

Materials

- Smartphone or tablet with Internet access
- Cards from the **Educator Resource: Linking Sexuality and Technology,** created prior to the session
- **Handout: Parental Values about Technology Use**
- **Handout: Online Resources for Teenagers**
- **Handout: On the Same Side: Family Agreement about Staying Safe Online**
- Optional: Signs labeled **Agree** and **Disagree,** posted on opposite walls

Procedure

1. Welcome the group. If you have not already been introduced by the program's sponsor, say a few words about your professional background, and provide an overview about the goals for the program, which are as follows:

   a. State that one would be hard pressed to find two more interesting and relevant issues for teens than SEX and TECHNOLOGY. **It is safe to say that many adolescents are preoccupied with both!** Explain that you are going to begin the program by providing examples about how sexual issues work their way into the technological arena.

   b. The next part of the program is designed to explore the balance between **protecting** teens from some of the dangers inherent in technology use, as opposed to **exposing** adolescents to online resources that promote safety, health and well-being. Emphasize that not everything about technology use is harmful or dangerous.

   c. Lastly, we are going to review a questionnaire that members in a family can complete at home. The questionnaire is designed to establish a set of safety standards that all agree are mutually beneficial.

2. Randomly distribute the cards from the **Educator Resource: Linking Sexuality and Technology** throughout the group. Ask the participants to take turns reading their examples out loud. This will set the tone for group participation early in the program. Use the questions listed below to process the activity:

   Discussion Questions:

   a. What are some of your reactions to the ways in which teens are linking sex with technology?

   b. If you read between the lines, what can these examples tell us about the physical, emotional and social challenges that teens are experiencing?

   c. Which of the examples did you find challenging as a parent? Why?

   d. Did any of the examples illustrate how technology might benefit the health and well-being of adolescents? In what ways?

3. Conclude this activity by pointing out that adolescent sexual development is a complex process that takes place over a number of years. Teens must adjust to their changing appearance, heightened sexual sensations, sexual attractions and social standing, and most importantly, must emerge from the process with a sense of normalcy. **The examples we read illustrate how teenagers are using technology as a means for understanding their own sexual development.**

4. In this next exercise, parents are introduced to some of the possible choices that they might confront when dealing with the challenges of the digital age.

   Distribute the **Handout: Parental Values about Technology Use,** and ask the participants to pair up with a person nearby to complete the task that is outlined.

   Alternative procedure:
   If you have the space and the group is small enough, draw an imaginary continuum down the center of the room. At one end, place a sign labeled **Agree,** and at the other end, **Disagree.** As you read each of the items on the **Handout: Parental Values about Technology Use**, ask the participants to stand at a point on the line that best represents their opinion about that issue. Participants should stand in the center when they are **Unsure** about how to respond. Read the items slowly, allowing time for the participants to share the reasons behind their chosen options.

   Regardless of which format is used, emphasize that there are no right or wrong answers to any of the items that will be explored. The purpose of the exercise is to open up new ways of thinking by exchanging ideas with one another.

5. When the exercise is completed, reconvene and process with a discussion:

   Discussion Questions:

   a. Which items evoked definite, clear-cut responses on your part? Why?

   b. Which items were challenging? Why?

   c. Did you learn anything new to think about from one another?

   d. Did you change your mind about anything as you participated in this exercise?

   e. Do you believe that technology is making our kids more casual about sex, or more promiscuous? Explain.

   Conclude by stating that contrary to popular belief, increased exposure to sex-related information in the digital age has not resulted in greater promiscuity or irresponsibility. The Centers for Disease Control and Prevention (CDC), has been reporting record lows in teenage pregnancy among women aged 15-19. Teens seem to be less sexually active, and more of those who are sexually active use birth control than in previous years.[1]

---

[1] Centers for Disease Control and Prevention. (2013). Teen pregnancy: The importance of prevention. Retrieved July 24, 2014 from http://www.cdc.gov/teenpregnancy

6. This portion of the lesson raises awareness about sexual health websites for adolescents. The idea of exposing teens to such resources will be new for many parents, and some may be uncomfortable with the idea of candid sexual health information at their children's fingertips. Tell participants they will have an opportunity to critically examine and decide which websites they feel comfortable recommending for their children.

7. Distribute the **Handout: Online Resources for Teenagers** and allow a few minutes for the participants to read it silently. Follow up with a discussion:

    Discussion Questions:

    a. As you were growing up, what resources did you turn to for sex-related information? Were books on sexual topics made available by your parents?

    b. Have any of you ever logged on to a sexual health website for teens? If so, what was your impression about the site and the information that was offered?

    c. What are some of your concerns about exposing teens to sex-related information? What are the potential benefits of providing teens with accurate information?

    d. When you look at the examples of the types of questions that can be found on sex-related websites, what do you think teens are looking for? How do you feel about their questions? Are your children asking similar questions?

    e. Do you think you might want to endorse and recommend specific online resources that you believe would benefit your child?

    f. If you decided to recommend a website that you believed was beneficial, what kind of message would you be sending to your child?

8. This portion of the lesson addresses online safety. Since safety issues are generally foremost on parents' minds, the participants will evaluate a tool that families can use at home when discussing online safety. Distribute one copy of the **Handout: On the Same Side: Family Agreement about Staying Safe Online** to each participant. Divide the participants into small groups, or ask them to pair up with a person sitting nearby. Their task is to critically evaluate the handout.

    Allow time for the participants to review the handout, and follow up with a discussion.

Discussion Questions:

    a.   What are some of your opinions about the handout?

    b.   Were you familiar with the safety recommendations that were listed on the handout? Were any of the recommendations new or different from the ones you already know?

    c.   Would you add any recommendations to the list?

    d.   Do you think that this would be an effective tool for your family to use? Why, or why not?

    e.   Do you have other ideas about how families might address online safety?

9.   The conclusion of this lesson illustrates how technology can benefit **parents.** Ask volunteers to use their smartphones (or have an extra phone or tablet on hand) to search for information using the following terms:

- **online safety tips for teenagers**
- **parents talking to teens about pornography**
- **parents talking to teens about sexting**
- **teenagers and cyberbullying**

Ask the volunteers to read some of the sites that their searches uncovered. If your location does not have Internet access, suggest that parents search at home, using these terms, or others of interest. Suggest that when searching for information, read selectively until appropriate material is located.

End the lesson with a message of support for parents. Just as technology can benefit the sexual development of adolescents, parents now have access to information that simplifies and clarifies how to engage in constructive conversations about sexual issues. All the help and support a parent might need in meeting the sex-related challenges of adolescence is just a click away!

Linking Sexuality and Technology

All of the examples listed below demonstrate how teens link their sexual interests and concerns with technology use. Copy and distribute the statements throughout the group, and without interruption, ask the participants to read the examples out loud. This is a way to open up many issues for discussion, without presenting information in a lecture format.

---

1. I sleep with my cellphone on my pillow in case my boyfriend calls. My mother wants me to leave my phone in the kitchen at night. She has no idea how important this is to me.

---

4. I keep asking my girlfriend to send a nude picture. She keeps telling me "no."

---

2. I Googled "how to put on a condom" and was surprised at the number of sites I found.

---

5. I was playing a game online, and a porn pic came on the screen! I wasn't even searching for it.

---

3. I like a website where you can ask the questions that you have about sex, and they will tell you the answers. You can also find out what other people are asking.

---

6. I'm gay and get bullied a lot in school, and now I'm being bullied on Facebook. I only feel I can be myself when I go into a chat room for kids who are like me.

---

7. My parents had a fit when they saw a pic of kids making out at a party on my Facebook page. Would that seriously prevent anyone from getting a job twenty years from now?

10. A boy in my class posted a pic of me on his Facebook wall, with a caption calling me a "slut." I've never even had sex yet.

8. My father told me that he didn't want me looking at porn. When I said that it was my business, he took away my cellphone because it didn't have blocks on it. Now I watch porn at my friend's house.

11. I'm overweight, so now I go on a website that gives tips on how to improve your self-image.

9. I took a pic of myself wearing a new outfit, and posted it on Instagram. Kids from school began letting me know whether they thought I looked good or not. I cried so hard, I didn't want to go to school the next day.

12. I wonder whether you can get herpes from kissing someone who has a cold sore. I better look that up.

Parental Values about Technology Use

Directions: For each item, check the box that best describes your opinion.

	Agree	Disagree	Unsure
1. No electronic devices should be allowed at the dinner table.			
2. Blocking sexual content on computers is an important protective measure.			
3. Socially isolated teens can benefit from interacting with others online.			
4. Watching pornography in moderation is not necessarily harmful.			
5. I would rather my child search for information about birth control or sexually transmitted infections than risk unwanted pregnancy or disease.			
6. Electronic devices should be placed in the common areas of the home, where parents can monitor their use.			
7. Instagram, an app for exchanging photos with friends, is a good form of social networking.			
8. I have been successful at restricting violent video games.			
9. Parents should definitely become a "friend" on their child's social networking account.			
10. Parents are as addicted to technology as are their kids.			
11. The sites that answer children's questions about sex lead to early sexual experimentation.			
12. My child might be more inclined to ask sex-related questions online than to ask me directly.			

Online Resources for Teenagers

The journal *Clinical Pediatrics* published a study evaluating different sexual health information websites for adolescents.[1] Eight of the highest scoring websites are listed below.

> **www.plannedparenthood.org**
>
> **www.scarleteen.com**
>
> **www.avert.org**
>
> **www.pamf.org/teen**
>
> **www.sexetc.org**
>
> **www.youngwomenshealth.org**
>
> **www.nhs.uk/livewell/sexandyoungpeople**
>
> **www.kidshealth.org**

The information found on these websites is provided or monitored by professionals with backgrounds in medicine and human sexuality. On these sites, adolescents can search for specific information and review answers to questions that are raised by others; on the sites that contain blogs, they can express their own opinions. The types of issues addressed include body image, sexual orientation, sexual decision making, birth control, sexually transmitted infections, relationships, abuse, consent, etc. Questions are answered honestly and openly.

A few examples of the types of questions raised on these sites are listed below:
> **How do I let go of feeling sexually unattractive?**
> **Sex hurts my girlfriend. How do I fix it?**
> **Is it normal for an ejaculate to look thick?**
> **Does porn influence your sexuality?**
> **How can you tell if you are gay or lesbian?**

Begin by visiting some of the recommended websites. Many parents find this to be an invaluable experience. The sites address a wide range of teenage sexual concerns, which are especially eye-opening for parents who grew up in a time when access to sexual information was limited. Observing the ways in which the professionals respond to commonly asked questions is often instructional for parents who are developing their own communication skills. After completing a review, you will be better equipped to decide whether you want to introduce your child to any of the recommended websites.

---

[1] Whiteley, L. B., Mello, J., Hunt, O., & Brown, L. K. (2012). A review of sexual health web sites for adolescents. *Clinical Pediatrics, 51(3):* 209-213.

On the Same Side:
Family Agreement about Staying Safe Online

Directions: Staying safe online is in every member of your family's best interest. As you work together to review each of the safety recommendations listed below, do the following:

- Discuss whether you agree with the recommendation.
- Give examples that show how you might benefit from following the recommendation.
- Feel free to revise, cross out or add recommendations. **Come up with a list that works for your family!**

✓ Nothing is private in cyberspace. If you don't want people all over the world to see what you are about to transmit, think twice before sending it.

✓ Once you transmit something over the Internet, understand that you can never take it back, even if you delete it. This is because others can copy and re-post, or save to their own devices, etc.

✓ Never transmit anything that might harm, embarrass or spread false rumors about others.

✓ Install safety controls on all of the social media accounts used by members in your family. For example, if you want a Facebook profile to be sent only to your "friends," not to their "friends" too, adjust safety controls to limit the spread of personal information. Check your accounts for instructions about how to install safety controls.

✓ Never give out your name, address or phone number to unknown people online.

✓ Never agree to answer sexual questions, send nude photos or meet offline with unknown people who contact you on social media.

✓ Do not send pictures that can prove to be embarrassing, now or in the future. Sexually suggestive poses or pictures that are made in fun can present the wrong impression if ever viewed by classmates, teachers, college admissions officers or future employers.

✓ Never lend or walk away from your phone or computer without standing nearby to observe how your electronic device is being used. Never give out your password; enter it yourself. When an electronic device is left unattended, remember to log out.

HELPING TEENS ACT PURPOSEFULLY IN A DIGITAL WORLD
A Lesson for Parents and Professionals

By Lee Heerten, MSW[*]

Objectives
By the end of this lesson, participants will be able to:

1. Recognize the psychological and social needs being fulfilled through youth's digital interactions.

2. Formulate ways to facilitate healthier digital interactions to fulfill youth's needs.

Rationale
Parents and youth-serving professionals are inundated with media reports of youth behaving badly online — stories of cyberstalking, sexting and cyberbullying can lead many caring adults to wish that youth would leave digital life altogether. However, as digital spaces and interactions have become seamlessly integrated into many young people's lives, they can also be powerful sites for young people's psychological and social needs to be fulfilled. This lesson encourages caring adults to recognize the possible motivations behind young people's problematic digital interactions, affirm the real and complex needs of youth, and assist young people in finding healthier ways to fulfill their needs, both online and off.

Materials
- Flip chart paper or board, markers
- Paper and pens or pencils
- **Educator Resource: Know Your Needs** (see Volume I, pages 15-18)
- **Educator Resource: Scenarios** (see Volume I, pages 19-20)
- **Educator Resource: Fact Sheet** (see Volume I, pages 21-22)
- **Handout: Understanding and Addressing Digital Dilemmas**
- **Optional:** Tape and pieces of paper each labeled with one of the psychological and social needs identified in the lesson

---

[*] Lee Heerten, MSW, is a wellness educator – sexual health at the University Health Center at the University of Nebraska – Lincoln.

Procedure

1. Introduce the lesson by asking participants if while watching a youth's behavior they have ever asked themselves, "Why on earth would they do that?!" Invite participants to share examples of young people's seemingly idiosyncratic or strange behaviors (but be careful to maintain an environment that is youth-positive, not disparaging). Acknowledge that youth sometimes act in ways that don't readily make sense, and that this can be frustrating for caring adults who want to see youth make positive, constructive choices in their lives.

2. Explain that humans are complicated and messy creatures — we don't always understand why people act the way they do, youth and adults alike. However, if we know the *intentions* or *motivations*, we can begin to better understand the actions. Some of the most basic motivators are our *needs*.

3. Explain that a need is anything that is essential and necessary for life, growth and well-being. Tell participants that they'll be exploring specific types of needs in this lesson: psychological and social needs. Psychological needs exist inside of us and we fulfill them through our own feelings, thoughts and behaviors. Social needs exist between us and other people and we fulfill them through our interactions with other people.

4. Distribute a **Need, Definition** or **Statement** card from the **Educator Resource: Know Your Needs** to each of the participants. Instruct participants to form small groups with others who have the complementary need, definitions or statements. Inform participants of how many people will be in each group once they have found each other. Caution participants that some of the definitions or statements may seem like they could apply to more than one need. They should keep in mind the difference between psychological and social needs and work together to come to a consensus.

Alternative Step:

Post pieces of paper labeled with each of the psychological and social needs around the room. Distribute a **Definition** or **Statement** card from the **Educator Resource: Know Your Needs** to each of the participants. Instruct participants to gather under the need that best matches their definition or statement. Have participants share their definitions and statements with each other.

Note:

The alternative step may work better for larger groups where several participants may have the same definition or statement or for groups where you are unable to anticipate the number of participants.

5. Once small groups have formed, distribute paper and pens or pencils. Instruct each group to select the definition that they believe best explains the need or to come up with a new definition that incorporates the best from each definition or statement. Ask participants to brainstorm with their small group some of the ways that young people fulfill this need in their lives. Have each

group share their need and definition, along with a couple of examples of how this need can be fulfilled, with the larger group.

6. Highlight any examples groups gave that utilize technology. If no group mentioned an example that involved technology, point out that, in addition to the examples they gave, many young people are increasingly using technology to try to fulfill these needs. Ask for any examples participants have of youth using technology to fulfill needs.

   ### Discussion Questions:

   a. What sort of role should caring adults play in helping youth fulfill their psychological and social needs? How does this role change based on the need or the relationship with the youth?

   b. Why do you think teens are turning to technology to fulfill these needs?

   c. Do you believe that technology is a generally effective or generally ineffective way for youth to fulfill their needs? Why?

   d. Do you think *your* relationship with technology impacts your view of how youth should be interacting with technology? In what ways?

7. Tell participants that they will now have an opportunity to help some hypothetical young people fulfill their needs. Explain that they will be given a scenario that a young person might face. In small groups they will try to find other ways the young person can fulfill their needs. Offer to work through one scenario together as a large group.

8. Select one of the scenarios from the **Educator Resource: Scenarios** to read, or have a volunteer read, to the large group.

   ### Discussion Questions:

   a. Were the interactions in this scenario familiar to you? From your experiences, what would be a more common or realistic scenario?

   b. What need or needs do you think the youth in the scenario was trying to fulfill?

   c. What was problematic or unhealthy about the way the youth was using technology to attempt to fulfill their needs?

    d. What are some healthier or less problematic ways, with or without technology, the youth could fulfill their needs?

    e. What are ways that a caring parent or professional could help a youth fulfill these needs?

9. Give each group a scenario from the **Educator Resource: Scenarios** and a copy of **Handout: Understanding and Addressing Digital Dilemmas.** You may need to re-divide participants into new small groups depending on the number of scenarios you use. Ask participants to answer the same questions as above in their small groups. Encourage participants to rewrite the scenario, if necessary, to reflect their experiences or interactions with youth and technology. Once groups have completed their discussions, ask each group to read their scenario to the rest of the participants and report back on their discussion. Give opportunities for participants to comment on other groups' scenarios.

You can refer to the **Educator Resource: Fact Sheet** for information about each scenario.

Discussion Questions:

    a. How did you feel about the young people in these scenarios?

    b. Did understanding the need motivating their behavior affect how you felt?

    c. What can caring adults do to help make young people more aware of the psychological and social needs they're trying to fulfill?

    d. Thinking of your children or the young people you work with, how do you think they would react to your suggestions for alternative behaviors? Are there any suggestions or strategies for making them more receptive?

    e. Is there anything that you're considering doing differently in your interactions with young people after this lesson?

Understanding and Addressing Digital Dilemmas

Directions: Read your scenario and, as a group, discuss and answer the following questions.

1. Were the interactions in this scenario familiar to you? _____

2. From your experiences, what would be a more common or realistic scenario?

   _____

   _____

   _____

   _____

   _____

3. What need or needs do you think the youth in the scenario was trying to fulfill?

   _____

   _____

4. What was problematic or unhealthy about the way the youth was using technology to attempt to fulfill their needs?

   _____

   _____

   _____

5. What are some healthier or less problematic ways, with or without technology the youth could fulfill their needs?

   _____

   _____

   _____

6. What are ways that a caring parent or professional could help a youth fulfill these needs?

_____

_____

_____

_____

_____

A 21ST-CENTURY CONVERSATION GUIDE TO TEENAGE SEXUALITY AND TECHNOLOGY
A Lesson for Adults

By Shanna M. Dusablon Drone, MSW, MAEd, MEd[*]

Objectives
By the end of the lesson, participants will be able to:

1. Identify at least three social media platforms (Facebook, Twitter, Reddit, Instagram, Snapchat, etc.) teens use for the exchange of sexual communication.

2. Practice communication skills regarding the intersection of sexuality and technology with consent, boundaries and legal consequences.

3. Practice communication skills concerning teen sexuality and technology.

Rationale
Adolescents use social media for sexual communication with little thought for the positive and negative results of using this medium. Adult caregivers including parents, social workers and other youth-serving professionals are key stakeholders in guiding adolescents into learning decision-making skills about sexual communication through various social media. Social workers and probation officers are included in this group due to the high-risk behaviors in which some adolescents take part that may result in negative legal or social consequences. Adolescents and their adult caregivers may struggle in communicating about sexuality topics in general (e.g., birth control, safer sex practices and STIs/HIV); the addition of sexual communication through social media adds another dimension to conversations that may further hinder their success. This lesson aims to empower adults as well as increase their comfort levels regarding communication skills in reference to adolescent sexuality and technology.

Materials
- Flip chart paper or board, black and colored markers
- Index cards with different stickers/pictures (Prepare prior to activity: Affix a sticker to an index card and then affix the same type of sticker to another index card, e.g., two index cards, each with a yellow star; two index cards, each with a red star, etc. There should be enough "matching pairs" according to your participant count.)

---

[*] Shanna M. Dusablon Drone, MSW, MAEd, MEd, is a sexuality educator with W.R.a.P. It Up – Sexuality Education With Respect and Purpose, based out of Victorville, CA.

- Title three sheets of flip chart paper as follows and post around the room:

      CONSENT – 1   **BOUNDARIES – 2**   **LEGAL CONSEQUENCES – 3**

- **Handout: Table Conversation**
- **Handout: Starting "The Talk"**

Procedure

1. As a large-group discussion, prompt the participants by asking the following:

    Discussion Questions:

    a. What is social media?

    b. What are examples of social media? (*List the participant answers on the board/flip chart. Examples may include Facebook, Instagram, Snapchat, Twitter, etc.*)

    c. How many of you have an account with some form of social media?

2. Have participants get into small groups, and distribute the **Handout: Table Conversation.** Have them discuss the questions with their group for about five to ten minutes.

3. Ask table members to report back on the questions from their table for a whole-group discussion.

4. Thank the participants for their insights about teens and social media. Explain that they are now going to move on to an activity that looks at consent, boundary issues and legal consequences.

5. Point to the various flip chart papers hanging up around the room. Inform participants that they will break up into small groups to discuss what issues they think are associated with each concept and how they relate to teen sexual communication.

6. Have the participants number off from one to three. Direct them to go to the paper that coordinates with their number.

7. As participants are gathering and moving toward their pieces of flip chart paper, walk around and pass out a marker to each group.

8. Inform the participants that they will have approximately three to five minutes in front of each flip chart paper to write down as many issues related to the concept (consent, boundary issues and legal consequences) and to teen sexual communication. Explain that once the time is up, you will pause the activity and ask the groups to move to the next sheet to the right."

9. Give each group approximately three to five minutes with each piece of flip chart paper to discuss and write their answers. After the time passes, ask the groups to move to the right again. Repeat this until each group has a chance to work with all three papers.

10. After participants have completed writing their answers to all three concepts, direct participants back to their seats. Collect the markers from each group as they walk back to their seats.

11. Read the responses out loud and ask for any clarifications if necessary.

    Discussion Questions:

    a. Do you notice any similarities among the answers?

    b. Do you notice any differences among the answers?

    c. Which issues strike you as especially important? Why?

12. Inform participants that these are the working issues for the next activity.

13. Pass out the index cards with stickers. Explain that there is a sticker on each card and that two people in the group have the same sticker. Each participant should find the person who has the matching sticker, introduce themselves and sit next to each other.

14. Ask the participants to raise their hands if they remember their parents having "The Talk" with them about sex. Ask if anyone is willing to share how that conversation went or felt.

    Note:
    As the educator, feel free to share a story from your own experiences as you see fit. Sharing a personal story allows for the educator to connect on a personal level with the participants, therefore creating and contributing to the group.

Discussion Questions:

a. Was there something you wish an adult had said or done differently regarding the conversation about sexuality?

b. What is a conversation you are most proud about having, either as a teen or adult, regarding sexuality?

15. Acknowledge that as an adult in today's world, sexuality may still be a difficult topic to discuss with a teen. While some people may be great at it, others may experience anxiety about how to handle the conversation. But in this fast-paced world of technology, those conversations are more important than ever to have with teens.

16. Explain that the participants *are going to practice talking about sex!* In this exercise they are going to role-play being an adult and a teen having a conversation about teen sexuality communication using social media.

17. Distribute the **Handout: Starting "The Talk."** Explain that the handout includes several conversational prompts for an adult and teen concerning the use of social media to communicate about sexuality, focusing on the issues of consent, boundaries and legal consequences.

18. Participants will have three rounds to practice talking about these issues. In the first round, one person should play the role of the adult and the other partner should play the role of the teen. For the second round, switch roles. In the last round, discuss what it was like to practice these conversations. Think about the reality of having these conversations with your teen.

Discussion Questions:

a. By a show of hands, how many think you would be comfortable talking with your teen about sexuality and technology?

b. What do you think would be difficult about the conversation and these issues?

a. What do you think would be positive about having these conversations?

19. Explain that they will have five to ten minutes for each conversation. Inform them that when the time is up, you will call out to move on to the next conversation.

20. Once the participants are clear on what they are expected to do, allow them to begin role-playing.

21. Allow five to ten minutes for each role play. Call out when it is time for them to move on to the next conversation. Inform participants that you will be walking around the room and are available for assistance if needed during this exercise

22. After the groups have done all three conversations, ask them the following questions:

    Discussion Questions:

    a. How did it feel to role-play?

    b. How might you use these conversations in your personal life?

    c. What are some other topics and questions you may have as either the adult or teenager based on the knowledge and communication skills you have practiced today? (*Direct their attention to the "Things to Remember" section of the handout.*)

    d. At the beginning of this activity, you were asked about your comfort level with this discussion. How many of you have increased your comfort level with this topic based on today's lesson?

23. Thank the participants for having this important conversation about social media and teen sexuality communication.

Table Conversation

Directions: At your table, discuss the following questions and be prepared to report back to the large group some key points about your table conversation.

1. How many of you know a teen who has an account on a social media site/app, or may have an account in the future?

2. How many of you are not sure if your teen has a social media account?

3. What do you think teens are communicating about in general using social media?

4. What do you think teens are communicating about regarding sex and sexuality, specifically, using social media?

Starting "The Talk"

Directions: During this activity, you will practice having a conversation about the topics of **boundaries**, **consent** and **legal consequences**. One of you will play the role of the adult, and one of you will play the role of the teenager. As the adult, read the prompt and then pick a question to start the conversation. Your "teenager" will respond with answers in a realistic way. Once you have completed one conversation in one of the three topics, switch roles and use the above directions to start the next conversation, moving from **boundaries** to **consent** to **legal consequences**.

If you are uncomfortable talking during this conversation, the following is a tip to ease into the conversation with writing:

- Ask the "adult" to write down the first thing they will say to the "teenager." Allow time to finish writing.
- Ask the "adult" to pass their handouts to the "teenager." Now the "teenager" will write what they think a "teenager" would say in response. Again, allow time to finish writing.
- Continue by having participants pass their handouts back and forth as the "adult" and "teenager" until the handout is completed.

Remember, this is your chance to feel more comfortable having these conversations, so take a deep breath and relax!

BOUNDARIES:

Getting Started

"I was reading our cellphone bill and noticed how much we all use our phones to surf the Web, text and take pictures, and all the different apps we use. I began to think about how much information is shared among you and your friends, partners and the Web."

Things You Might Want to Ask …

- o What information through text, picture or video do you think is OK to share with friends? Family?
- o What information do you think is not OK to share with friends? Family?
- o If you wondered if a text/picture/video was OK to share or look at, would you talk with someone about it first? Why or why not?

CONSENT:

Getting Started

"I read an article the other day about teenagers sharing naked pictures with each other through sites like Instagram. The article stressed some adults' concerns that these pictures are being shared without the knowledge or consent of the person in the picture."

Things You Might Want to Ask …
- o What do you think about pictures being shared without permission?
- o What would you do if you found out that someone shared any of your pictures without your permission?
- o How do you think this could happen?
- o Does it make a difference if the pictures are just of friends hanging out? If they are half-nude? Fully nude pictures? What do you think the difference is between these types pictures?
- o How can you be sure your pictures don't go out without your consent?

LEGAL CONSEQUENCES:

Getting Started

"In the news lately there has been a lot of information coming out about teenagers sexting. Some teenagers are being arrested for sharing and or viewing half-naked or naked pictures/videos of people."

Things You Might Want to Ask …
- o What does sexting mean to you? What do you think sexting means to other people?
- o What do you think about teenagers sharing these pictures? Is it OK for them to do that? Why or why not?
- o Do you know what the laws are concerning sexting in our county? When can we set up some time to research this area?

THINGS TO REMEMBER:

- • These **conversation starters** are intended to help make it easier for you to have conversations about sexuality and social media with your teen. Please feel free to modify according to the needs of your relationship with your teenager.

- • Talking about sexuality with your teen may occur spontaneously or be a planned conversation. You know what works best with your teen. Sometimes incorporating an activity such as cooking, walking, shopping or cleaning while having the conversation may help in increasing everyone's comfort level.

Resources Section

It's important for educators to be familiar with the technology and social media platforms that young people engage. The digital age is fast-moving and ever-changing, so this can be challenging!

This section contains a brief explanation and list of pros and cons of some of the most popular electronic tools and forums used by young people today. Included in this section are:

Apps

Clickers

Facebook

Controlling Your Privacy on Facebook

Instagram

Snapchat

Tumblr

Twitter

APPS

By Holly Moyseenko[*]

Background

The phrases *mobile applications* and *software applications* are often used interchangeably and are typically shortened to just *apps*. Apps are programs to help mobile devices (smartphones and tablets) do things — anything from email to games to social media to shopping. Apps are still relatively new, as the world first laid eyes on them in 2007, beginning on the iPhone and expanding to other smartphones. The Pew Internet Research Center reports that "[A]pp use has been a core feature in the broader move away from desktop computers toward mobile computing on handheld devices."[1] Apps have the ability to help offer the "promise of streamlining pager, cellular phone, Dictaphone and email messaging functions into a single device."[2]

Younger adults are more likely to use apps, and they tend to favor ones that allow them to stay in contact with others (for example, the type of apps they may prefer are texting, email and social media).[1] Smartphones allow for the technology to be wherever you are. While some apps are considered immensely vital for making life easier (for example, email apps), others exist purely for fun or utility (for example, games and shopping). One of the most popular types of apps, especially among adolescents and college-aged individuals, are social networking apps (e.g., Facebook, LinkedIn, Twitter, Tumblr and Instagram).

Advantages

- There are a significant number of free apps available.

- Some apps allow users to read, write and edit documents on a mobile device and transfer them back and forth to a computer (Quick Office and Documents To Go are two great options).

- Social networking apps can be useful to connect with others. A user can create groups on Facebook and LinkedIn for colleagues, individual classes, etc.

- Using apps in the classroom is a great way to be up to date.

- There are many apps that can be used in the classroom to encourage an interactive experience.

---

[*] Holly Moyseenko is a consultant for H & K Health.

[1] Purcell, K. (November 2, 2011). Half of adult cell phone owners have apps on their phones. Retrieved July 17, 2014 from http://www.pewinternet.org/2011/11/02/half-of-adult-cell-phone-owners-have-apps-on-their-phones/

[2] Adatia, F., & Bedard, P. L. (2013). "Palm reading": 2. Handheld software for physicians. *Canadian Medical Association Journal, 168(6):* 727-734.

Concerns

- Since anyone can create and release an app, there are no guarantees the app gives users accurate information.

- Some apps require a fee, and the fee does not necessarily guarantee quality. Users can navigate quality by reading others' app reviews.

- Some mobile devices may have limited storage, and thus will not be able to hold many apps at one time.

- If students use their mobile devices in class, it may be difficult to tell if they are using apps encouraged by the educator or if they are doing non-school related activities (for example, texting with their friends).

A Few Apps for Educators

- *Blackboard Mobile Learn:* Free for schools that utilize Blackboard; allows for users to check grades, assignments, discussion boards, etc.

- *Dropbox:* An app that allows users to store and access files "in the cloud" (the items are not stored on the device, but rather on a server). It is useful because the user can access their items from any mobile device or computer (that has the app installed), so it is a great back up, especially for conferences. Once you install or register, you will get 2GB of storage for free.

- *Google Drive:* A free app that allows users to store and access files "in the cloud." Users can also edit and add to any documents — some people use this as a way to keep track of communication with students or as a way to communicate with their colleagues. The Android version of the app has a slight edge as it allows users to "scan" a paper with their mobile device's camera.

- *Google Hangouts:* A free app that can be used as a digital way to hang out with others. This can be used to host meetings between different groups of people, as well as to chat with students.

- *Knowmia Teach:* A free app that can be used to create videos as well as view them. Users can create their own lesson, and allow students to both view the video created as well as post their own.

- *Nearpod:* An app that lets educators create and give presentations. Students can view the presentation, as well as take their own notes. Nearpod is more interactive than many similarly designed apps in that educators can add questions, polls, etc. to the presentation. The basic version is free.

- *Period Tracker:* A free app that allows the user to track her period, which can help forecast her fertility. The user can also add notes on her mood, any symptoms and intimacy. Can be useful to teach students about the menstrual cycle as well as the fertility awareness method of birth control.

- *PickMe:* An app that, with the press of a button, will randomly select the name of a student (and their picture, if you provide it) to call upon. The app costs $1.99, and you can even note if they answered correctly.

- *Schoology:* A free app that allows the educator to customize the experience for the students. Educators can create a space that students can access via a mobile device or using a computer that allows for discussion groups, due dates, the ability to send reminders, an easy way for students to turn in assignments, Dropbox, etc.

- *Socrative:* Both the educator and student versions of the app are free, and work together to create a dynamic classroom experience. Educators are able to ask questions using various formats (e.g., multiple choice, true or false, short answer) and students use their own mobile devices or computers to answer.

- *Splashtop:* An app that allows the user to remotely access their computer via a mobile device. Once the app is installed on the mobile device, the app will also need to be downloaded on the computer.

CLICKERS

By Susan Milstein, PhD, MCHES, CSE[*]

Background

There are many new technological tools that are now available for sexuality educators to use when designing and implementing their educational programs. One of the tools that have become available is an audience response system, often known as "clickers." Clickers are small handheld devices that allow students to respond to questions, and the results of the group can be instantly viewed on a graph that is generated within PowerPoint. Clickers can be used in traditional classroom settings, and they can also be a part of community-based educational efforts.

Clickers can serve a variety of purposes, including identifying class norms, addressing the issue of perceived norms, assessing current knowledge levels of participants, and being able to get an instant understanding of participants' beliefs on a variety of personal topics relating to sexuality. There are different brands of clickers, including Turning Technologies and iClicker.

Alternatives to Clickers

Recently, online polling systems, such as www.polleverywhere.com, have become available. These systems offer many of the same benefits of clickers, but do not require any specific hardware. Educators may create polling questions online and poll their audiences using any computer that has access to the Internet. People can respond to a variety of polls, such as True/False questions and open-ended questions, using their smartphones.

Advantages

- Everyone can participate, even those who are afraid of sharing their thoughts out loud. Because clickers can be used anonymously, this technology allows people to be able to share their opinions, without fear of being judged.

- Clickers allow the educator to quickly check comprehension! If participants need to know specific information in order to be able to move on to the next part of a lesson or activity, a clicker question or two can quickly allow the educator to see how much the participants know, and if they're ready to move on to the next step.

- Clickers are PowerPoint-based. If an educator is familiar with PowerPoint they will be able to easily create and implement presentations that use clickers.

---

[*] Susan Milstein, PhD, MCHES, CSE is the founder and lead consultant of Milstein Health Consulting.

- Using clickers helps make the learning experience more personal. Educators may rely on national statistics in their presentations and participants may not feel that those numbers apply to them or the people they know. Asking questions by clicker allows everyone to see how the statistics in the room compare to those national numbers, which may make the information more relevant.

Concerns

- Results may be unexpected. Educators who use clickers will need to be able to think quickly on their feet, as the answers to questions may be surprising!

- Clickers may not be cost effective. While they can be a great teaching tool, there is a cost associated with clickers that can range into the hundreds of dollars depending on how many an educator needs to purchase. Online polling systems offer a cheap, or sometimes free, alternative. The cost is often determined by how many people will be responding to each question.

- Technology doesn't always work the way we hope. An educator may design a great clicker presentation, but if the display for the PowerPoint isn't working then the presentation may be useless. Similarly, if an educator is using an online polling system, they must have reliable Internet access or else the polling cannot work.

FACEBOOK

By Timaree Schmit, PhD[*]

Background

Facebook is by far the world's largest social media site, with over 170 million users in the United States alone and nearly 1.3 billion worldwide. Among people who use the Internet, 72% have Facebook accounts.[1]

Facebook has a wider variety of applications than any other social media site, enabling users to create personalized profiles that can be connected to others; post lengthy text, images, and videos; join public and private special interest groups; "like" and respond to each other's content; share messages and events; and check in at locations and occasions to let others know where they are. Groups, businesses and organizations can create pages used to share content and interact with fans and customers. Users can "friend" each other to connect profiles and users can "like" pages to follow its posts. Profiles are also used as identity verification for registering with other sites and apps.

While nearly every racial and economic demographic uses the site, slightly more females than males do. Young adults between 18 and 30 are the heaviest users[1] but adults aged 45-55 are the fastest growing membership group.[2]

Advantages

Potentially, Facebook can be used to reach the widest possible audience through both organically grown social connections and paid advertisements. With the variety of applications, sexuality educators can foster an active and engaged community by posting things of interest and encouraging interactive comment threads in response. It's a one-stop shop for events promotion and incredibly easy to navigate.

Concerns

While Facebook dominates the Internet and has become almost as standard as email or a telephone for communication, it has lost a great deal of its cool cachet among young people. While profiles and newsfeeds can be personalized to limit who sees what, many teens and tweens are reluctant to use a site that is also frequented by their parents and grandparents. This demographic is sometimes better

---

[*] Timaree Schmit, PhD., is a sexuality educator, host of "Sex with Timaree" podcast, and professor of Human Sexuality at Widener University and Community College of Philadelphia.

[1] Smith, C. (June 24, 2014). By the numbers: 125 amazing Facebook user statistics. Retrieved July 16, 2014 from
http://expandedramblings.com/index.php/by-the-numbers-17-amazing-facebook-stats/#.U8boY4zD9LM

[2] Cooper, B. B. 10 surprising social media statistics that might make you rethink your social strategy. Retrieved July 16, 2014 from https://blog.bufferapp.com/10-surprising-social-media-statistics-that-will-make-you-rethink-your-strategy

accessed through media like Twitter, Instagram and Snapchat. It's best for educators who are working with young people to routinely ask their students about what apps are popular and how they work.

Sex educators specifically need to be aware of the censorship imposed by Facebook's Community Guidelines. While frowned upon, violence is far more accepted on the site than sexuality, especially nudity. Posting depictions of nipples or genitalia can result in a profile or page being temporarily disabled or even permanently deleted. So use images with caution and encourage students to be contemplative before posting them as well.

Best Practices

It's important to balance personal and professional personas to retain boundaries with students and clients. Be mindful of who can see what; make use of the settings to filter what is published. Consider having a private personal profile for friends and family and a public professional page to engage with a wider audience. Interact regularly with other people's posts; Facebook rewards what they call "heavy users" by promoting their content to the top of friends' newsfeeds.

By learning the nuances of the site, user engagement can be maximized. Know the time of day your target audience is most likely to use the site. Include images whenever possible to increase attention, either by posting pictures and videos or simply by making sure a link includes a thumbnail. Posts should be frequent to maximize exposure (at least five a day), but spaced apart by a minimum of an hour. They can be scheduled to post ahead of time, so there is no need to spend the entire day in front of the computer to be consistently engaging. Tagging can be used to alert specific people and organizations about content that is relevant to them and to boost the signal of any given post. Ask open-ended and thought-provoking questions that will encourage interaction and reward users for their efforts by "liking" thoughtful comments and responding to them. Make sure to review for copyediting before posting.

CONTROLLING YOUR PRIVACY ON FACEBOOK

By Josefina Gil-Leyva[*]

Your Facebook posts might not be as private as you thought they were. Facebook has settings you should become familiar with in order to control your privacy. There are some posts you cannot make private, e.g., your cover photo and any comment you make on a post that is visible to everyone.

Privacy Settings and Tools

Facebook has a section called "Privacy Settings and Tools" where you can control the privacy of your posts, albums, who can contact you, etc. It would be a good idea to visit the Help Center where privacy settings are explained in detail. (Click "Help" at the bottom of the Facebook login page, or if you are logged in, click the "down arrow" in the upper right then click "Help.")

Facebook gives you the option of making posts, albums and sections of your page visible to everyone, friends, friends of friends, a specific group of friends, or only yourself. Keep in mind that once you change the privacy settings on a post, the next post will keep the same privacy setting as the last one. Check the settings before posting; you also have the option of editing a setting after posting.

Timeline and Profile Visibility

On your profile page, from the "View Activity Log" drop-down menu located at the right of your cover photo, select the "View As…" option. This will show you how your Timeline looks to others who are not your friends on Facebook. Keep in mind that Facebook is constantly making changes to its look and settings. It would be a good idea to use the "View As…" setting to see how your profile looks to everyone.

Tagged Photos of You

Even though you can make your photos private, friends of friends — or everyone — can see a tagged photo of you, depending on the photo's privacy settings. If someone tags you in a photo that is visible to everyone, then everyone will be able to see it and will also have the link to your Facebook page. You have the option of removing the tag or asking the person to remove the photo. You can find the "Remove Tag" option at the bottom of each picture under the "Options" label.

Graph Search

Facebook recently added "Graph Search," where you can type "photos of [name]" into the search bar, including the name of the person of whose photos you want to see. This means anyone who is

---

[*] Josefina Gil-Leyva is a health educator at Planned Parenthood of Central and Greater Northern New Jersey.

not on your friends list will be able to look up photos in which you are tagged or that you posted that are visible to everyone. If you don't want your photos to be public, make sure you set the privacy settings on each album to "friends only"; there are some albums where you can change the audience for each photo.

Who Can Find You

You have the option of letting everyone, friends of friends, or only friends find your Facebook page using your phone number or email address. This means anyone who has this information can look you up unless you make it private. Phone apps have the ability to find the Facebook pages of all of the contacts saved on a phone but you can control how easy it is for someone to find your page. You also have the option of changing the privacy of your phone number and email address so that nobody can see them, or only friends, or everyone.

INSTAGRAM

By Holly Moyseenko[*]

Background

Instagram was introduced in October 2010[1] as an application (app) that allowed users to share pictures. The app regularly updates, allowing for new features. It allows users to edit photos using various filters, for different finishes that give the pictures different appearances. The filters can give the picture a "Photoshopped" look with a few quick taps, and no knowledge of editing required. Through the platform, users may also share their photos on other social media sites (for example, Facebook, Twitter, Tumblr, etc). Most people under the age of 22 have grown up with technology all around them, and many are already using (or at least familiar with) social media. As of spring 2014, Instagram is the preferred social network among teens.[2] By using Instagram in the classroom, you're meeting students where they already are!

Getting started is easy as long as you have access to a smartphone or tablet. Simply download the Instagram app, then create an account. Once an account is created, you can take photos using the Instagram app or use photos already on the device. If you prefer to not use your phone, you currently will not be able to post photos, but you can still follow accounts, comment and "like" pictures. You can create an account by going to http://bit.ly/InstagramAccountAndUsername.

Once you create your account it is useful to create a bio, which you can do by going to "Edit Your Profile." Shorter and succinct tends to be better. You can search for users that you know, or simply search using different hashtags. (More about hashtags at right.) If you find someone you would like to follow, simply click the blue "Follow" button below their profile picture. This person will now show up in your feed — but your pictures will not show up in theirs unless they follow you. Users may "like" and comment on other users' pictures. When you post a new picture, you can choose to include

What's a Hashtag?

Hashtags are clickable links that can help to engage users, as well as connect you to new users. Hashtags are easy to use — just type # and (without any spaces) any word or phrase that you think describes the picture or will help link people to what you are trying to say or show (e.g., #condoms). Many educators will create a hashtag of their last name or the name of the class or workshop to help students easily follow along and contribute. Instagram has a very active Community Team, which creates different projects to engage users. One of the most popular is the "Weekend Hashtag Project" which has a new theme each weekend. Users are encouraged to participate (they are often sent a text message, if they included a way for Instagram to contact them) using that weekend's hashtag.

---

[*] Holly Moyseenko is a consultant for H & K Health.
[1] Instagram. (n.d.). Our story. Retrieved July 17, 2014 from www.instagram.com/press
[2] Piper Jaffray. (Spring 2014.) Taking stock with teens: A collaborative consumer insights project. Retrieved July 18, 2014 from http://www.piperjaffray.com/private/pdf/Taking_Stock_Teach-In_Spring_2014.pdf

just the picture itself, any number of hashtags, any number of words, or any number of words and hashtags.

Instagram can be used to interact with students and other sex educators.[3] The social networking app is useful for conferences — possibly by using a common hashtag, as often done using Twitter. It can also be used as an engagement tool, not just by sharing pictures but especially by interacting with other users by re-posting their pictures and commenting.[4] One blogger on education suggests that Instagram can be used as "a great tool to teach digital etiquette... an avenue to connect with educators and students from around the state, nation, and world... [and] documentation of all the amazing learning activities that occur."[5] If you want students to create accounts, it is best to familiarize yourself with Instagram's Terms of Use (for example, currently users must be at least age 13 to create an account, although people of any age may view Instagram).

Advantages

- Very user friendly. College-aged students and younger have always had technology, and the vast majority is already using social media.

- There is the ability to make your account "private" so that you will need to approve another user in order for them to be able to view your photo stream. This can be useful if you want to keep your personal Instagram account.

- Users can decide if they want to share any commentary with their photo or let their pictures speak for themselves.

- Since sex education isn't just in a classroom, Instagram makes it easy to share anything related to sex education when found out "in the wild."

- Users can choose to include their location (known as "geotagging") on individual photos, as well as whether or not to tag other users in each picture. Users can then click on the location to view other pictures from that location.

- Using a catchy picture or a picture of a short sentence is great for getting the attention of other users, then including a link to a site or blog.

- Social media in general is fantastic for making students more engaged. Ashley MacQuarrie, an online community manager, suggests that "students may be more engaged in their work

---

[3] Salomon, D. (2013). Moving on from Facebook: Using Instagram to connect with undergraduates and engage in teaching and learning. *College & Research Libraries News, 74(8):* 408-412.

[4] Shouse, S. (October 23, 2013). Instagram for higher education. Retrieved July 17, 2014 from http://visionpointmarketing.com/blog/entry/instagram-for-higher-education

[5] James, J. (July 10, 2013). Invitation: Instagram for educators. Retrieved July 17, 2014 from http://currentsofmyriver.blogspot.com.au/2013/07/invitation-instagram-for-educators.html

---

when they feel they have an *authentic audience* — that someone other than their teachers will see it. Just as with blogging and tweeting, Instagram is a social sharing application, so the authentic audience is definitely there."[6]

Concerns

- Anyone can post any picture. There is no verification process.

- You cannot directly post pictures from a computer at this time, but anyone can still view the Instagram site, comment, and "like" pictures.

- It's not possible at this point to share or re-post a picture using the Instagram app — you will need to upload the picture yourself then post or use another app (such as InstaRepost or Repost for Instagram).

- A smartphone or tablet is required to easily post photos.

- While users can edit any photo that they upload, if you are into more advanced editing, you may get bored easily with the options.

- While Instagram is very user friendly, if you aren't very familiar with technology and apps, there may be a bit of a learning curve.

---

[6] MacQuarrie, A. (November 20, 2012). Using Instagram as a learning opportunity. Retrieved July 17, 2014 from http://blog.k12.com/educational-technology-and-tools/instagram-education#.UuUE1NIo7s0

SNAPCHAT

By Corbin Knight-Dixon, MS[*]

"This message will self-destruct in five seconds." A self-destructing message was once an object in spy series and films — today it exists as a popular photo-messaging application ("app") that can be downloaded onto your smartphone. Snapchat, first developed in 2011, is an app that allows its user to take pictures and send them to other Snapchat users. With over 100 million reported users, Snapchat has become a popular and controversial social media platform.

The Basics:

- Take a snap — a photo or video that can be edited and sent to recipients on your "My Friends" list.
    - Tap the screen to snap a photo or press and hold to take a video snap.
    - Caption your photo or video using the pen tool or caption text boxes.

- Time how long your message to be seen by the recipient before it "self-destructs." Snaps cannot be longer than 10 seconds.

- Send your snap by selected one or more friends. The status of the Snapchat can be viewed on the dashboard.

- View your snap easily. You'll receive a notification in your Snapchat dashboard when you have a new message. Once you click on the message, you can view the content that was sent to you for the period of time determined by the sender.

- Chat by sending a message or photo to others (similar to a SMS or text message) or video chat in real time. Like snaps, these messages "self-destruct" after being viewed by the receiver of the message.

- Share your story. Snapchat makes sharing a private photo or video snap easy. It is just as easy to publicize a snap to your friends by adding it to your story, a series of snaps that create a narrative. Once added, your Snapchat friends can view the snap an unlimited number of times for 24 hours.

Pros:

- Novelty: Snapchat is one of the newest and more popular social media platforms for young people aged 13-24.

---

[*] Corbin Knight-Dixon, MS is the sexual health program coordinator for Harlem RBI.

- Privacy: Although controversial, many users report that they feel their content is safe when sent via Snapchat instead of a text message. The app also has a notification that warns the user if their snap has been made into a screenshot.

- "Who Can Send Me Snaps": Snapchat privacy settings allow users to limit who they receive snaps from to friends only.

- Support: Snapchat has a built-in support system that allows the user to report any harassment or violation.

Cons:

- Privacy: There has been debate whether an image can be deleted forever. Many in the field of cyber forensics argue that digital images such as snaps cannot be permanently deleted.

- Security: Users who allow content from "Everyone" are exposed to higher risk from unwarranted outside Snapchatters.

- Sexually explicit snaps: There has been great concern about "sexting" among minors using the Snapchat app and about what other explicit content they are able to send virtually.

- Reporting: While Snapchat allows its users to report harassment, the fact that the content erases itself may cause senders to communicate more explicit or brash content.

TUMBLR

By Corbin Knight-Dixon, MS[*]

Background

With nearly 200 million blogs,[25] Tumblr has quickly become one of the most diverse social media platforms on the Web today. Tumblr allows the user to publish a wide variety of content including text, photos, quotes, links, chats, audio and video. Gone are the times of verbose text posts via blogging websites — Tumblr is a whole new way to share information and tell your story.

Tumblr provides many social features. Once an individual creates an account they have the ability to post content, follow blogs, ask the blog owner questions and reply to and "like" individual posts.

How to Use Tumblr

Create a Tumblr by:

- *Signing up:* Joining Tumblr is free and requires an email address, password and your age. You must be at least 13 years old to create a new Tumblr blog.

- *Making a username:* Your newly created username will double as your URL, so if your username is "safersex4all", your URL will become www.safersex4all.tumblr.com. The URL must be unique to the Tumblr universe, which is no easy feat with nearly 200 million registered blogs.

- *"Tell us about yourself":* Tumblr will prompt you to add a picture, title the blog and provide a description. All of these will be public on your blog but can be edited at any time.

- *Navigating the dashboard:* The Tumblr dashboard is the mission-control center for your new blog. It allows you to post content, see recent posts for the blogs you follow, view account details and much more!

Start "tumblogging" by posting to share your story in a multitude of ways:

- *Text:* Includes a title and text block which has a wide variety of formatting options such as adding hyperlinks or images.

- *Photo:* Upload up to 10 photos from your computer along with a caption. For easy uploading, users can also copy and paste an image's URL from the Web.

---

[*] Corbin Knight-Dixon, MS is the sexual health program coordinator for Harlem RBI.
[25] Tumblr. (n.d.). Press information. Retrieved August 16, 2014 from http://www.tumblr.com/press

- *Quote:* Publish a quote and its source to your blog. No need to add quotations or hyphens within the post, Tumblr will take care of all the specific formatting for you.

- *Link:* Highlight an important link by inputting its URL, a link title and caption (optional).

- *Chat:* Share previous conversations or online chats by following Tumblr's specific formatting instructions. This feature is not a way to live chat with other Tumblr users.

- *Audio:* Upload audio content from your computer, a website URL, or from popular platforms such as Spotify or SoundCloud.

- *Video:* Upload a video from your computer or copy and paste a video's embed code or URL from popular sites like YouTube.

- *Social features:* Connect and engage with new people worldwide.
  - *Follow:* Similar to Twitter, following on Tumblr will add the blog to your dashboard and allow you to keep up with another user's most recent posts. To follow a blog go to their personal page and click the "Follow" button in the top right hand corner.
  - *Reblog:* If another user submitted something you would like to add to your Tumblr, select the "Reblog" button, add any additional content Tumblr will allow, and then publish the post.
  - *Like:* See something you like but do not want to add to your Tumblr? Click the heart button to "like" the post. Likes also operate similarly to bookmarks which can be accessed from your dashboard.
  - *Reply/Message/Ask:* Tumblr's additional social features allow you to communicate with a blogger privately.

Advantages

- *Tag your content:* Add a hashtag to all of your posts and give other bloggers the ability to search tags for posts that may apply to their interest.

- *Queue and draft posts:* Just like a draft email, you can save a draft post and edit it at a later date. Queuing a submission will save posts and publish them over a period of hours or days based upon your specifications.

- *"There's an app for that":* Connect easily to your Tumblr dashboard from your smartphone or tablet.

- *Anonymous questions:* Bloggers have the option of allowing their viewers to post questions or comments anonymously. This allows followers to ask questions without fear of judgment.

Concerns

- *Anonymous questions:* Anonymity can lead to bullying or harassment of a Tumblr user. Individuals can "Ignore" messages to permanently block public or anonymous users from submitting messages and are encouraged to contact Tumblr's support team to report abuse.

- *Privacy:* Tumblr is primarily a public platform and does not allow individuals to filter who is able to view their content. Users can explore additional privacy options and policies at http://www.tumblr.com/about.

- *Explicit content:* Tumblr supports bloggers in publishing content that is explicit but requires them to flag their blogs as Not Safe for Work. Users can filter out NSFW blogs from their dashboards.

TWITTER

By Timaree Schmit, PhD[*]

Background

Twitter is a social networking site and microblogging platform with 255 monthly active users,[1] including many celebrities with whom regular people can interact directly. Users create and post tweets that are limited to 140 characters, but can also include images and links to external content. It is one of the top 10 most-visited sites on the Web[2] and over 500 million tweets are generated every day.[3] Of all adult Internet users, 19% use Twitter.[4] Users are likely to be younger than 30.[5] For teens and tweens, Twitter is a close second to Instagram as the preferred social networking site, pulling ahead of Facebook since 2013.[6]

Advantages

Due to its simplicity, Twitter is incredibly easy to use. It allows for instantaneous sharing of current events and facilitates conversations between individuals who would otherwise be strangers. While users can "follow" others whose posts they want to see, no commitment is required to interact with other public profiles. Hashtags can used to cultivate conversations about specific topics and boost the signal of specific posts while tagging and private messages are used to notify other users directly (see p. 121 for further explanation of hashtags). Interesting content can be both "favorited" and re-shared with one's followers in the form of a retweet. While text is limited in length, space-saving acronyms are common and links will point readers to longer stories. There is almost no oversight of the content, so censorship of sexual content is not a concern.

Concerns

The 140-character maximum is notoriously challenging to in-depth or nuanced discussions. Conversations between users are not presented in thread form, which can make it harder for readers to follow. Lack of community standards or oversight means there are few mechanisms for preventing harassment and bullying. Classroom discussions on Twitter should also focus on discretion and

---

[*] Timaree Schmit, PhD., is a sexuality educator, host of the "Sex with Timaree" podcast, and professor of Human Sexuality at Widener University and Community College of Philadelphia.

[1] Twitter. (n.d.). Company. Retrieved July 18, 2014 from https://about.twitter.com/company

[2] Wikipedia. (June 25, 2014). List of most popular websites. Retrieved July 18, 2014 from
   http://en.wikipedia.org/wiki/List_of_most_popular_websites

[3] Twitter. (n.d.). Company. Retrieved July 18, 2014 from https://about.twitter.com/company

[4] Pew Research Center. (January 2014). Social networking fact sheet. Retrieved July 18, 2014 from
   http://www.pewinternet.org/fact-sheets/social-networking-fact-sheet

[5] Hindenbach, J. (August 27, 2013). Adults vs. teens: How we use social media. Retrieved July 18, 2014 from
   http://www.nextadvisor.com/blog/2013/08/27/adults-vs-teens-how-we-use-social-media

[6] Piper Jaffray. (Spring 2014.) Taking stock with teens: A collaborative consumer insights project. Retrieved July 18 from
   http://www.piperjaffray.com/private/pdf/Taking_Stock_Teach-In_Spring_2014.pdf

privacy. Make use of examples from the news of inappropriate tweets that had real-world consequences; discuss reasons for setting one's feed to private.

Best Practices

The best tweets are simple, direct and interesting. Spend time crafting tweets for succinctness, clarity and wit. Writing original content will drive more followers, but retweets are an important way to build community and can foster relationships among users who share interests. By being aware of common and trending hashtags, users can reach a wider audience. Hashtags can also save valuable characters by providing instant context for posts. Twitter works best for real-time interactions and tweet chats can be organized and promoted in advance to bring people together at a set time to talk about an issue, connected by a hashtag.

To make it easier to organize one's Twitter feed, people that a user follows can be organized into lists by theme, subject matter or other category. One good use of lists is "Follow Friday," denoted by hashtag **#FF**. It's a tradition on Friday for users to post suggestions for other people of interest to follow. **#FF** is most effective when all the suggested people have a common thread connecting them: shared expertise, geography, etc. **#FF** can be helpful in cultivating relationships with people who are more famous or influential in a given field, as it serves as a cross-promotion of their posts and of the others who are suggested.

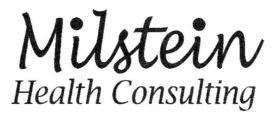

Milstein Health Consulting

● ● ● ● ● ● ● ● ● ● ● ● ● ● ● ● ● ●

Milstein Health Consulting was created to help meet your health information needs. Our presentations, workshops, and "lunch and learns" are designed to provide practical, science-based health information for your high school, college, business, or community group.

We offer consultation on a variety of health topics. If you don't see what you're looking for, contact us and we'll create a presentation or workshop to meet your needs.

Presentations and Workshops

Sexuality
Topics include:
- Ask the Sexpert ... a Q&A workshop
- HIV and STIs: The basics
- Contraception 101
- Sexuality and aging
- Healthy relationships …. for all ages

Workshops for Parents
- Teen sexuality
- Teens and body image

General Health
Topics include:
- Stress management
- Body image
- Nutrition
- Fitness
- Weight management
- Men's health
- Sport performance
- Approaches to alcohol and other drugs

● ● ● ● ● ● ● ● ● ● ● ● ● ● ● ● ● ●

For more information:

www.milsteinhc.com

info@milsteinhc.com
240-498-8823

HAVE ONE OF OUR
SEX ED
TRAINERS AT
YOUR NEXT EVENT!

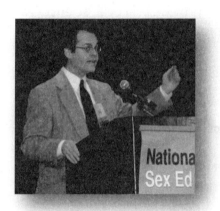

Our nationally known trainers present **workshops** and deliver **keynote addresses** that help professionals teach about safer sex and other sexual health topics.

Attendees leave our programs empowered with the skills and confidence to teach sex ed. (Plus ready-to-use lessons!)

Our trainers have many years of experience providing sexuality education in an array of settings, and are widely respected as leaders in the field.

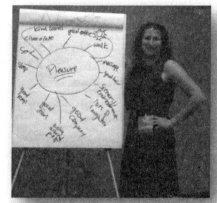

To arrange a speaker at your next event, please contact
(973) 387-5161 or email
Info@SexEdCenter.org

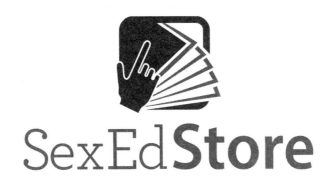

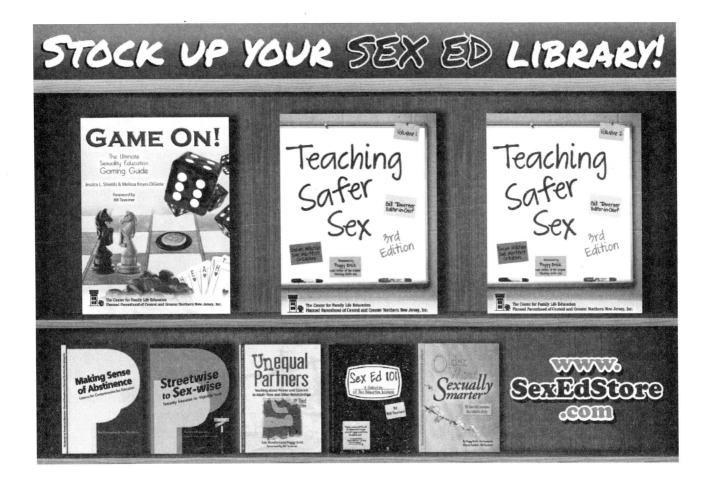

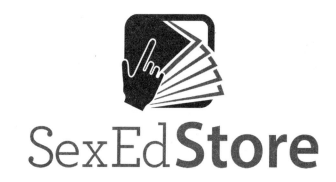

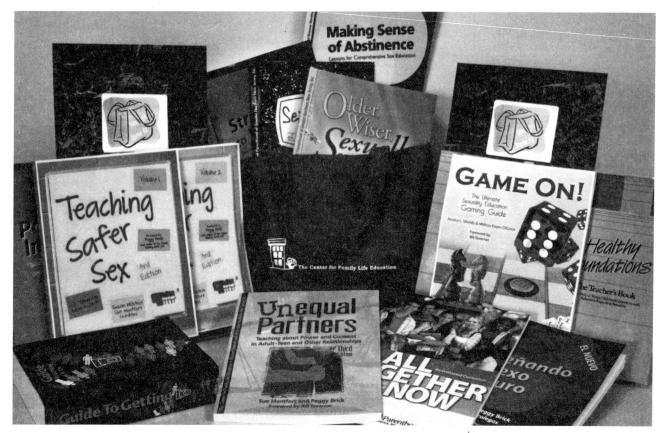

SEX ED DELUXE KIT

The **Sex Ed Deluxe Kit** includes all the publications by the CSE, plus a few other surprises for teaching about sexuality through the lifespan! Ideal for new educators to be fully equipped with a complete library of lessons! Great for veteran educators replenishing their resources!

This set of books that retails "a la carte" at almost $800 is available for

$499

plus shipping.

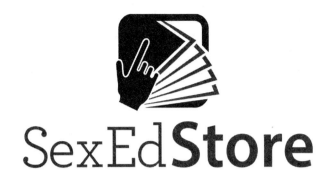

SexEd**Store**

All Together Now
An evaluated curriculum with five favorite lessons for teaching about contraception and safer sex

Changes, Changes, Changes! Great Methods for Puberty Education
Features nine chapters with more than 40 engaging and informative lesson activities

Educating About Abortion, 2nd Edition
10 lessons to help students examine the facts and their own beliefs about abortion

Enseñando el Sexo Seguro
20 lessons for teaching safer sex in Spanish, developed in cooperation with MexFam and reviewed for cultural competency

Game On! The Ultimate Sexuality Education Gaming Guide
20 amazing lessons and activities for engaging your students' learning through gaming

Healthy Foundations Series
Includes three books: **Bodies, Birth and Babies,** providing background and sample training modules; **Healthy Foundations – The Teacher's Book,** to help respond to young children's questions and behaviors about sexuality and **Healthy Foundations – Developing Policies,** to help pre-schools and child-care centers develop sexuality policies and programs

Making Sense of Abstinence
16 positive lessons for teaching about abstinence in the context of comprehensive sex education

Older, Wiser, Sexually Smarter
30 sex ed lessons for older adults

Positive Encounters: A Guidebook for Professionals
An essential guidebook for positive one-to-one interactions with teens about contraceptive and safer-sex decisions

Positive Images, 4th Edition
35 lessons for teaching about contraception and sexual health

Sex Ed 101: A Collection of Sex Education Lessons
10 popular lessons spanning a wide range of sexual health topics.

Sex Ed in the Digital Age, Volumes 1 & 2
30 lessons designed to equip parents, educators, and students with skills that are necessary for meeting the challenges of addressing sexual health in the digital age

Streetwise to Sex-Wise, 2nd Edition
Two series of lessons for teaching about sexuality to high-risk youth

Teaching Safer Sex, 3rd Edition, Volumes 1 & 2
50 great lessons – 25 in each volume – for teaching about sexual safety

Unequal Partners, 3rd Edition
30 lessons for teaching about power and consent in adult–teen and other relationships

ORDER FORM

Name:_____

Daytime Phone:_____

Email:_____

Organization:_____

Address:_____

City:_____ State:_____ Zip:_____

TITLE	QUANTITY	PRICE	SUBTOTAL
All Together Now	_____	@ $49.00	_____
Changes, Changes, Changes	_____	@ $69.00	_____
Educating About Abortion, 2nd Ed.	_____	@ $39.00	_____
Enseñando el Sexo Seguro	_____	@ $49.00	_____
Game On!	_____	@ $69.00	_____
Healthy Foundations Series (3 books)	_____	@ $39.00	_____
Making Sense of Abstinence	_____	@ $39.00	_____
Older, Wiser, Sexually Smarter	_____	@ $49.00	_____
Positive Encounters: Guidebook	_____	@ $29.00	_____
Positive Images, 4th Ed.	_____	@ $69.00	_____
Sex Ed 101	_____	@ $39.00	_____
Sex Ed in the Digital Age, Vols. 1 & 2	_____	@ $99.00	_____
Streetwise to Sex-Wise, 2nd Edition	_____	@ $49.00	_____
Teaching Safer Sex, 3rd Ed., Vols. 1 & 2	_____	@ $99.00	_____
Unequal Partners, 3rd Ed.	_____	@ $59.00	_____
*Sex Ed Deluxe Kit (all this and more!)**	_____	@ $499.00	_____

Add $8.00 s/h for first item; $2.00 for EACH additional item _____

Add $30.00 s/h for Sex Ed Deluxe Kit

TOTAL ENCLOSED: _____

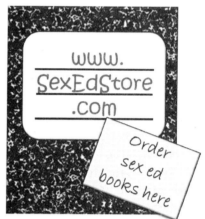

If your order is above $500, please contact us at Info@SexEdCenter.org for bulk-order pricing.

Please make checks payable to:
PPCGNNJ
196 Speedwell Avenue
Morristown, NJ 07960

Phone: (973) 387-5161
Fax: (973) 539-3828
E-mail: Info@SexEdCenter.org

For credit card orders, check one:
____American Express ____Discover
____MasterCard   ____Visa

No.: _____

_____

Expiration Date _____

Signature:

_____